Pitfalls in Prescribing and How to Avoid Them

Pitfalls in Prescribing and How to Avoid Them

HUGH McGAVOCK BSc MD FRCGP
Visiting Professor of Prescribing Science
Department of Nursing Studies, University of
Ulster and Course Organiser, GP Continuing
Clinical Education, Northern Ireland Medical
and Dental Training Agency

Radcliffe Publishing
Oxford • New York

Radcliffe Publishing Ltd
18 Marcham Road
Abingdon
Oxon OX14 1AA
United Kingdom

www.radcliffe-oxford.com
Electronic catalogue and worldwide online ordering facility.

British Library Cataloguing in Publication Data

A catalogue record for this book is available from the British Library.

New research and clinical experience can result in changes in treatment and drug therapy. Readers of this book should therefore check the most recent product information on any drug they may prescribe to ensure they are complying with the manufacturer's recommendations concerning dosage, the method and duration of administration, and contraindications. Neither the publisher nor the author accept liability for any injury or damage arising from this publication.

1005970835

ISBN-13: 978 1 84619 332 3

Typeset by Pindar NZ, Auckland, New Zealand
Printed and bound by TJI Digital, Padstow, Cornwall, UK

Contents

To Elizabeth, my companion in medicine and life.

Introduction

Fifty years ago, medicinal drugs were mostly weakly effective and relatively non-toxic in prescribed doses. Today's clinician has therapeutic powers which our predecessors half a century ago would have considered miraculous in their effectiveness and in the range of diseases that can now be prevented, cured or their progress slowed. Together with this power for therapeutic good there has been an undeniable risk of drug-induced harm, through inappropriate use or dosage, side-effects, drug–drug interactions, failing metabolism in the liver and reduced excretion by the kidneys. Erratic compliance with drug taking by a large proportion of patients complicates and sometimes worsens iatrogenic harm.

The sad fact is that preventable prescription-related disease (PPRD) is common throughout the developed world. In general practice (primary care), much PPRD goes unrecognised and unrecorded. Proof of its existence is provided by comprehensive research in many western countries which shows that between 3% and 5% of all Accident and Emergency (A & E) admissions are directly caused by prescribed medicines. This figure rises alarmingly to around 12% of all elderly emergency A & E admissions. In hospital, too, PPRD is common, often due to dosage and administration errors, and hospitals now employ clinical pharmacists to assist in and monitor the prescribing and administration of medicines.

All prescribers should be aware of these statistics, for without realising it, they may be part of the problem. That need not be. This book offers the clinician the knowledge with which to avoid the commonest pitfalls in prescribing. Except where it is essential to clear understanding, 'fancy science' has been omitted, or made immediately accessible. The book is intended primarily for family doctors who on a daily basis must prescribe a wide range of drugs, including regimens recommended by specialists. Many specialist nurse practitioners and independent nurse prescribers should also find this book a helpful exposé of prescribing pitfalls and a guide to safer prescribing. *Pitfalls in Prescribing* should be very useful in the tricky process of medication review now required by the Quality and Outcomes Framework (QoF) for GPs in the United Kingdom.

A series of clinical scenarios illustrating prescribing pitfalls is included at the end of the book. Enthusiasts may wish to self-test on these cases before and after studying the book's contents!

1

1

Treatment failure due to antacids

Complex modern drugs have a variety of chemical radicals which readily interact with other compounds in the body. Indeed, it is just such properties which enable drugs to bind to their intended target to achieve their therapeutic effect (*see How Drugs Work*, Chapters 5 to 9).[1] Unfortunately, a number of important drugs react chemically with all antacids containing calcium, aluminium or magnesium, if any of these are present in the stomach or duodenum when the drug is swallowed. This reaction alters the drug's structure and either prevents its absorption from the intestine or renders it inactive at its target site in the body – heart, liver, kidneys, etc. The inevitable result is therapeutic failure, and unless you are aware of its cause, you will not recognise the problems. Table 1.1 lists the most important drugs which must not be taken if there is antacid in the stomach. From this you will realise how important the problem is. Many clinicians are unaware of the risk, and since antacids are so widely consumed by patients who 'don't think it worth mentioning' to the doctor or nurse, the problem needs determined action to prevent it.

TABLE 1.1 Drugs whose absorption is impaired if an antacid has been taken

DRUGS OR DRUG GROUPS	Result of interaction with antacid
ACE inhibitors	Poor control of hypertension
Antibiotics: azithromycin, ciprofloxacin, isoniazid, rifampicin and most tetracyclines, etc.	Infection does not respond to treatment
The antivirals, amprenavir, atazanavir, tipranavir	Infection does not respond to treatment
The antifungals itraconazole and ketoconazole	Infection does not respond to treatment
The anti-epileptics phenytoin and gabapentin	Risk of seizures
The phenothiazine antipsychotics and sulpiride	Recurrence of psychotic symptoms
The anti-malarials: chloroquine, hydroxychloroquine and proguanil	Failure of anti-malarial protection
The bisphosphonates	Failure of osteoporotic therapy
digoxin	Treatment failure
oral iron	Anaemia fails to respond
lansoprazole	Failure of ulcer or GORD treatment
The antihistamine fexofenadine	Symptoms unrelieved
dipyridamole	Reduction in prophylactic effect
rosuvastatin	Failure of lipid lowering

GORD, gastro-oesophageal reflux disease; *See* also *British National Formulary (BNF)*, Appendix 1: Antacids.[2]

In the light of Table 1.1, it is clearly essential that prescribers warn patients not to take antacids just before or at the same time as their prescription drugs. Pharmacists, too, need to reinforce this message at every repeat dispensing, and to ask patients about prescription drugs whenever they sell an antacid over the counter (OTC). If the drugs in Table 1.1 are taken before a meal, there is no reason why an antacid, if needed, should not be taken *after* the meal, when it will not affect drug absorption.

For those curious enough to wish to know the antacid–drug interaction involved, there are four:
1   formation of a chemical complex – complexation
2   adsorption of the drug by the antacid
3   resin binding

4 destruction of a drug's acid-resistant coating due to the increased pH in the stomach that results from the antacid.

So next time you encounter treatment failure, don't increase the dose without asking the following questions:
1 Is it due to non-compliance?
2 Is it due to an antacid?

REFERENCES
1 McGavock H. *How Drugs Work*. 2nd ed. Oxford: Radcliffe Publishing; 2005.
2 Joint Formulary Committee. *British National Formulary*. 56th ed. London: British Medical Association and Royal Pharmaceutical Society of Great Britain; 2008.

2

2

Grapefruit juice can cause drug toxicity

As every clinician knows, the small intestine is not just a passive membrane. A major part of its complex function is the active absorption of nutrients, salts and some vitamins. What many people still don't know is that the small intestine also has a powerful drug-metabolising mechanism whose evolutionary function was to detoxify poisonous materials ingested with food, preventing their absorption and rendering them harmless. This mechanism includes enzymes identical to the drug-metabolising liver enzymes – the so-called cytochrome P_{450} oxidase system (of which more in Chapter 9).

Unfortunately for the prescriber, these enzymes in the intestinal mucosa also metabolise and render impotent many important modern drugs, of which the left column of Table 2.1 is a major sample. Drug companies are well aware of this, and set the standard dose of the drugs shown in Table 2.1 up to double the dose that would be adequate were the intestine devoid of metabolic function. So what is the problem? It is that a single glass of grapefruit juice, half a grapefruit or a Seville-type (bitter) orange irreversibly blocks the intestinal P_{450} enzymes for up to 24 hours. During that period, up to double the correct dose of the drugs in Table 2.1 may be absorbed into the circulation. This may lead to toxic concentrations in the tissues. Note that it doesn't matter at what time the grapefruit juice is consumed – the intestinal metabolic enzymes will be 'knocked out' for 24 hours. Some authorities, who should know better, suggest that a litre of grapefruit juice must be consumed to cause this effect. This is not so – a 250-ml glass is enough to affect the intestinal enzymes as described.

TABLE 2.1 Drugs whose absorption is enhanced by a glass of grapefruit juice, a helping of grapefruit or a Seville (bitter) orange

Drug(s) or drug group	Result of enhanced absorption
Calcium-channel blockers – all except diltiazem	Hypotension with all. Risk of heart block and heart failure as well, with verapamil
amiodarone (see Chapter 3 for its many risks)	Risk of circulatory collapse and hepatic toxicity. See BNF
simvastatin and atorvastatin	Increased risk of liver toxicity and side-effects
All erection-enhancing drugs	Hypotension, priapism and other side-effects
Immunosuppressants – ciclosporin, sirolimus and tacrolimus	Irreversible rejection of grafted tissue
Antivirals – efavirenz and saquinavir	Failure to control the infection
warfarin	Enhanced anti-coagulation and its risks
The anxiolytic buspirone	Excessive and prolonged sedation
carbamazepine	Risk of blood, liver and skin disorders (see 24 lines of side-effects in BNF Chapter 4.8.1)
sertraline	Risk of hypotension, tachycardia, confusion, amnesia, aggression and serious liver and pancreatic disorders

See also British National Formulary (BNF), Appendix 1.

TACTICS TO AVOID THE RISK OF EXCESSIVE DRUG ABSORPTION

1 *The Easy Way Out (EWO)!* The simplest way of avoiding the risks of grapefruit juice is to tell all patients taking short-term or maintenance medication to avoid it. This is no great hardship, and a 'blunderbuss' approach makes life a little easier for the prescriber and the dispenser.

2 *A more subtle tactic.* Use your prescribing software to 'flag up' a warning message on the counterfoil of the prescription form, whenever one of the drugs listed in Table 2.1 is prescribed. This should always be accompanied by a strong verbal warning, since many patients don't read counterfoil instructions, let alone those on the patient information leaflet (package insert).

Have no illusions – grapefruit juice is a major prescribing pitfall, especially in older patients and those with reduced kidney or liver function.

For the curious, the culprit in grapefruit juice has been identified as a furanocoumarol, also found in bitter oranges. This blocks the intestinal P_{450} enzyme irreversibly. However, the intestinal mucosa generates a fresh population of enzyme, usually within 24 hours.

A footnote: cranberry juice

Cranberry juice enhances the anticoagulant effect of warfarin, and other coumarins, in some patients.

3

INTRODUCTION TO CHAPTERS 3, 4 AND 5: THREE EFFECTIVE AND DANGEROUS DRUGS

The following three important and commonly prescribed drugs, warfarin, amiodarone and all NSAIDs, are responsible for a disproportionate amount of preventable prescription-related disease (PPRD) and death – ask your local Accident and Emergency consultant! A large percentage of this drug-related harm is due to a failure to remember a few basic facts, and these chapters will aim to remind you of these.

3

Warfarin

Warfarin is a particularly effective drug in the prevention of deep vein thrombosis (DVT), pulmonary embolism, embolisation in atrial fibrillation and some prosthetic heart valves. It is also used during haemodialysis and to prevent myocardial infarction in patients with unstable angina. No better drug has been developed in the past 70 years. It was discovered and marketed by the Wisconsin Alumni Research Foundation as a result of their research into haemorrhagic disease in cattle, hence its name – 'WARF' plus 'arin', the last letters of coumarin, its chemical group. Its initial use was as rat poison. If you think of this every time you prescribe warfarin or co-prescribe it with another drug, you may avoid its becoming a human poison! As in rats, its main function is as a potent vitamin K antagonist, producing progressive, dose-related anticoagulation. As all family doctors and warfarin clinic nurses know, there is only a small difference between the clinically effective dose and the toxic dose, for a given patient. The maintenance dose must be determined for each patient by INR estimation, taken at the same time on each occasion and monitored regularly.

Every year, patients die as a result of being dispensed warfarin tablets 5 mg instead of the intended 0.5 mg (in hospitals as well as in primary care). This shouldn't happen. Prescribers who are aware of this possibility will regularly remind patients of their tablet colours – e.g. one *blue* tablet (3 mg) and one *white* tablet (0.5 mg) daily. This should be delivered verbally, written on the anticoagulation card and recorded in the patient's record. That simple ploy is doubly important if a carer is administering the drug; this includes residential and nursing homes, where the drug administrator may not have nursing qualifications.

However, the major cause of warfarin-related haemorrhage is its interaction with other drugs (*see* Chapter 9, and *How Drugs Work*, Chapter 23).[1] In each case in Table 3.1, the interacting drug potentiates warfarin – e.g. the anti-coagulation effect of warfarin is added to that of an NSAID (which may have been bought in a supermarket or convenience store). If the NSAID has caused a peptic ulcer, any gastrointestinal bleeding is likely to be severe and difficult to stop, because of the degree of anticoagulation by warfarin.

The drug interactions in Table 3.1 were identified as important in a long-term care setting in the USA, by the Medical Directors' Association. The 'culprits' are much the same in most countries' residential – and secondary – care sectors (*see* www.amda.com/m3).

TABLE 3.1 Important drug interactions with warfarin

Interacting drugs	Result of interaction
Warfarin and NSAIDs	High risk of profuse gastrointestinal bleeding
Warfarin and macrolides (e.g. erythromycin)	Potentiation of warfarin
Warfarin and quinolones (e.g. ciprofloxacin)	Potentiation of warfarin
Warfarin and phenytoin	Potentiation of effects of warfarin and phenytoin
Warfarin and amiodarone	Potentiation of warfarin

Every prescriber should memorise this short list – use the mnemonic 'NSAID – MACRO – QUINO – PHENO – AMIO.' Remember that these are only the commonest combinations that cause serious harm. The full picture can be found in the *British National Formulary (BNF)* Appendix 1, on the page of interactions with coumarins/warfarin. So if you are in any doubt, consult your *BNF* before issuing an 'add-on' prescription to any patient who is on a maintenance dose of warfarin.[2] Most UK pharmacists have high-grade drug interaction software and have the detailed pharmacological knowledge to use it effectively. They should warn you and the patient if they detect a significant risk. However, since – under the NHS – the dispensing pharmacist is not provided with a full medication list or even a diagnostic summary sheet, this excellent source of safety assurance may fail.

The alert reader will have noticed that warfarin was cited in Chapter 2 as one of the drugs whose absorption from the intestine is significantly enhanced by consuming grapefruit juice, grapefruit or bitter oranges within 24 hours. Ask yourself how many apparently poorly controlled 'anticoagulees' are drinking grapefruit juice. The family doctor and anticoagulation clinic nurse must warn them regularly and firmly to avoid this foodstuff.

Throughout this book, I shall cross-reference prescribing pitfalls. What better way is there to reinforce the messages?

REFERENCES

1 McGavock H. *How Drugs Work*. 2nd ed. Oxford: Radcliffe Publishing; 2005.
2 Joint Formulary Committee. *British National Formulary*. 56th ed. London: British Medical Association and Royal Pharmaceutical Society of Great Britain; 2008.

4

4

Amiodarone: a candidate for the title 'riskiest drug'

Amiodarone is a remarkably useful drug for treating cardiac arrhythmias. Its indications include atrial fibrillation and flutter, paroxysmal ventricular tachycardia, nodal and ventricular tachycardia, ventricular fibrillation and tachyarrhythmia. It is part of the management of many patients, greatly improving their quality of life and life expectancy. The *BNF* states that amiodarone 'should be initiated only under hospital or specialist supervision', and with very good reason.

This is because amiodarone presents the prescriber with two complex problems:

1 an unenviable list of adverse drug reactions (ADRs) due to amiodarone itself
2 an extensive and complex set of interactions with many other commonly used drugs – adverse drug interactions (ADIs).

Let us examine these problems separately.

THE ADVERSE DRUG REACTIONS (ADRS) OF AMIODARONE

Most family doctors know some of amiodarone's ADRs (e.g. phototoxicity and thyroid problems). Fewer prescribers are aware of all of them, and consequently the risks to the patient of lasting harm, with loss of quality of life and irreversible morbidity, are great. Most of these risks can be avoided if the problem is detected early by a knowledgeable prescriber or dispenser. **At this point it is worth noting that amiodarone's most serious ADRs will not manifest themselves as overt symptoms until it is too late. Their early presence will be detected only by specific symptomatic questioning by an informed doctor, nurse or pharmacist with a high index of suspicion.** When you have studied this short section, you will probably realise to what an extent such careful follow-up surveillance is our clinical responsibility. Table 4.1 summarises the main risks of amiodarone in monotherapy mode.

TABLE 4.1 The main ADRs of amiodarone and how to detect them at an early stage

Adverse drug reaction to amiodarone	Tactics for early detection by the prescriber
1 Pulmonary fibrosis, irreversible, often rapidly progressive and fatal. Mechanism unknown	1 Ask regularly about cough, wheeze or dyspnoea on exertion 2 Do regular pulmonary function tests 3 If suspicious, stop the drug, send for chest X-ray and refer to a specialist
2 Hypo- or hyperthyroidism. Amiodarone-induced hyperthyroidism may be refractory to treatment. Mechanisms unknown	1 Do TFTs six-monthly 2 *See BNF* for clear guidance on management
3 Hepatotoxicity	Do LFTs six-monthly
4 Ophthalmic ADRs: a. Corneal microdeposits (very common) b. Optic neuritis, leading to blindness. Mechanism unknown	a. Ask about 'glare' problems during night-time driving; it is *not* usually necessary to withdraw the drug b. Ask regularly about deterioration of daytime vision and use your Snellen's chart. A six-monthly check by an optometrist is advisable. If suspicious, stop the drug and refer as 'urgent – one week' to a retinal ophthalmic surgeon

(continued)

Adverse drug reaction to amiodarone	Tactics for early detection by the prescriber
5 Neurological damage – peripheral neuropathy or proximal muscle weakness	At each review, ask specifically about neurological symptoms – they may be trivial to begin with. If suspicious, refer urgently to a neurologist
6 Phototoxicity – the development of an irreversible, unsightly, purplish discolouration of all skin exposed to sunlight	Warn all patients to shield exposed skin and to use high-factor, wide-spectrum sun cream during treatment and for several months after stopping (amiodarone has a very long half-life – several weeks)

TFT, thyroid function test; LFT, liver function test.

Besides these relatively uncommon ADRs, by its known pharmacological actions on several organs, amiodarone is innately toxic for many patients. It is usually well tolerated in all but the highest doses. Unfortunately, the highest doses are used as 'loading doses' (necessary to achieve a 'steady-state' plasma concentration) in the first month of treatment. In high doses, and in patients whose drug metabolism is impaired, amiodarone is cardiotoxic, renotoxic and hepatotoxic. It acts particularly as a negative inotrope for the cardiac conducting system, but is a general myocardial depressant and will worsen congestive heart failure. In the kidney tubules, amiodarone reduces the excretion of basic (as distinct from acidic) drugs or metabolites. In addition to its inhibition of liver enzymes (described below), amiodarone in higher doses is a hepato-cellular toxin. It has the longest list of cautions, contra-indications and side effects of any *BNF* drug (*BNF* Chapter 2.3.2)

The *BNF*'s amiodarone monograph (*BNF* Chapter 2.3.2), is reproduced here, with the permission of the Joint Formulary Committee, British National Formulary 56 edn, London: BMJ Group and RPS Publishing; 2008, updated annually – consult the current edition at BNF.org.

'Amiodarone has a very long half-life (extending to several weeks) and only needs to be given once daily (but high doses may cause nausea unless divided). Many weeks or months may be required to achieve steady-state plasma-amiodarone concentration; this is particularly important when drug interactions are likely (*see also* Appendix 1).

Most patients taking amiodarone develop corneal microdeposits (reversible on withdrawal of treatment); these rarely interfere with vision, but drivers may be dazzled by headlights at night. However, if vision is impaired or optic neuritis or optic neuropathy occur, amiodarone must be stopped to prevent blindness and expert advice sought. Because of the possibility of phototoxic reactions, patients should be advised to shield the skin from light during treatment and for several months after discontinuing amiodarone; a wide spectrum sunscreen to protect against both long-wave ultraviolet and visible light should be used.

Amiodarone contains iodine and can cause disorders of thyroid function; both hypothyroidism and hyperthyroidism may occur. Clinical assessment alone is unreliable and laboratory tests should be performed before treatment and every 6 months. Thyroxine (T4) may be raised in the absence of hyperthyroidism; therefore tri-iodothyronine (T3), T4 and thyroid-stimulating hormone (thyrotrophin, TSH) should all be measured. A raised T3 and T4 with a very low or undetectable TSH concentration suggests the development of thyrotoxicosis. The thyrotoxicosis may be very refractory, and amiodarone should usually be withdrawn at least temporarily to help achieve control. Treatment with carbimazole may be required. Hypothyroidism can be treated with replacement therapy without withdrawing amiodarone if it is essential; careful supervision is required.

Pneumonitis should always be suspected if new or progressive shortness of breath or cough develops in a patient taking amiodarone. Fresh neurological symptoms should raise the possibility of peripheral neuropathy.

Amiodarone is also associated with hepatotoxicity and treatment should be discontinued if severe liver function abnormalities or clinical signs of liver disease develop.'

THE MAIN ADVERSE DRUG INTERACTIONS (ADIS) OF AMIODARONE WITH OTHER DRUGS

Before reading further, please study the large amiodarone drug interaction section, Appendix 1 at the back of the *BNF*). From this you may begin to wonder whether amiodarone should ever be prescribed, except as monotherapy! Of course it can be and should be, with acceptable risk, but only if the prescriber has an adequate understanding of its serious pitfalls, which the rest of this section will seek to reveal, as well as discussing how to side-step them.

What makes amiodarone so risky is that it exhibits *three distinct types* of potentially toxic drug–drug interaction. First, it inhibits the metabolism of a dozen important drugs (so-called pharmacokinetic interaction). Secondly, it interacts at the site of action or of therapeutic effect of a further dozen drugs (a pharmacodynamic action). Thirdly, it interferes with the renal excretion of several drugs, including lithium. We now need to look at each of these three interactions. They are collated in Tables 4.2, 4.3 and 4.4, with the main drugs with which amiodarone interacts. Their mechanism is included if known. All of these ought to be added to the practice prescribing software, so as to 'flag up' the possible interaction with amiodarone and to pre-empt harm to the patient and/or disruption of the treatment regimen.

Most doctors like a challenge! Here we have a most valuable drug which has not been superseded in 40 years. The challenge of its safe and effective use is more like a minefield than a series of pitfalls! It is hoped that this chapter will bring out in readers the clinical scientist of our highest aspirations.

GENERAL DESCRIPTION OF THE THREE AMIODARONE INTERACTIONS WITH OTHER DRUGS

1 Amiodarone inhibiting liver enzymes

In Chapter 2 we saw that amiodarone is one of the drugs whose absorption from the intestine is significantly increased due to the inhibition by grapefruit juice of drug-metabolising enzymes in the mucosa of the small intestine. This interaction can lead to toxic concentrations of amiodarone in the plasma. However, once in the bloodstream, amiodarone is itself a potent inhibitor of the liver metabolism of many common drugs. In the liver, amiodarone strongly inhibits several of the most important cytochrome P_{450} (CYP_{450}) metabolic enzymes responsible for the deactivation of many other drugs (*see How Drugs Work*, Chapter 3).[1] This leads to their accumulation in the body tissues and to the possibility of toxicity.

TABLE 4.2 Adverse liver interactions

Interaction	Drugs interacting	Nature of risks	Risk level
Metabolic enzymes in liver (CYP450) inhibited by amiodarone (*see How Drugs Work*, Chapter 3)	warfarin, phenindione	Plasma anticoagulant concentration rises ADJUST WARFARIN DOSE	High
	digoxin	Plasma digoxin concentration rises HALVE DIGOXIN DOSE	High
	phenytoin	Plasma phenytoin concentration rises	High
	ciclosporin	Plasma ciclosporin concentration rises	High
	eplerenone	Plasma eplerenone concentration rises	High
	flecainide	Increased risk of ventricular arrhythmias and T de P*	High
	procainamide and disopyramide	Increased risk of ventricular arrhythmias AVOID COMBINATION T de P*	High
Liver enzyme metabolism of amiodarone inhibited by:	amprenavir, nelfinavir, ritonavir	Plasma amiodarone concentration rises AVOID COMBINATION	High
	atazanavir	Plasma amiodarone concentration rises AVOID COMBINATION	High
	orlistat	Plasma amiodarone concentration rises AVOID COMBINATION	High
	cimetidine (often bought OTC)	Plasma amiodarone concentration rises AVOID COMBINATION	High

*T de P = torsade de pointes, a frequently fatal ventricular arrhythmia (*see* Chapter 7 for further details, including those most susceptible to it and therefore most likely to suffer this most severe drug-induced harm, i.e. women, and those with slow heart rate, myocardial disease, hypothyroidism, older age and electrolyte imbalance).

Table 4.2 shows the most serious of these interactions, adapted from Appendix 1 of the *BNF*.[2] The experienced prescriber will immediately realise why, in every case, the risk level is graded as 'high', for these are all drugs whose potential for toxicity is great and serious. In excess, warfarin, digoxin, phenytoin, ciclosporin, eplerenone and the antivirals are all dangerous. In addition, those drug–drug interactions in Table 4.2 and 4.3, liable to precipitate the frequently fatal ventricular arrhythmia known from its ECG appearance as 'torsade de pointes' (or 'twisted points'), are asterisked. Very briefly, this occurs after progressive lengthening of the cardiac action potential, measured by the QT interval of the ECG PQRST trace. It is a critical cardiological emergency. Those most likely to develop torsade de pointes are women, people with slow heart rate, those with preexisting myocardial disease or hypothyroidism, older patients, and those with drug-induced hypocalcaemia, hypokalaemia or hypomagnesaemia. If it happens to one of your patients, you are unlikely to forget it (*see* Chapter 7 for details).

2 Amiodarone augmenting the pharmacological action of other drugs

TABLE 4.3 Adverse interactions with amiodarone

Interaction	Drugs interacting	Nature of risk(s)	Risk level
Augmentation of pharmacological action of one or both drugs. Remember that amiodarone is a Class III anti-arrhythmic drug	All anti-arrhythmics (*see* also sotalol, diltiazem and verapamil below)	Increased myocardial depression and, in some cases, increased risk of ventricular arrhythmias (*see BNF*, Appendix 1: amiodarone) (T de P*)	High
	moxifloxacin	Increased risk of ventricular arrhythmias (T de P*) AVOID COMBINATION	High
	co-trimoxazole	Increased risk of ventricular arrhythmias (T de P*) AVOID COMBINATION	High
	Parenteral erythromycin	Increased risk of ventricular arrhythmias (T de P*) AVOID COMBINATION	High

(*continued*)

Interaction	Drugs interacting	Nature of risk(s)	Risk level
	clarithromycin	Increased risk of ventricular arrhythmias (T de P*) AVOID COMBINATION	High
	lithium	Increased risk of ventricular arrhythmias (T de P*) AVOID COMBINATION	High
	tricyclic antidepressants	Increased risk of ventricular arrhythmias (T de P*) AVOID COMBINATION	High
	mizolastine	Increased risk of ventricular arrhythmias (T de P*) AVOID COMBINATION	High
	Anti-malarials mefloquine, quinine, chloroquine, hydroxychloroquine, artemether/lumefantrine	Increased risk of ventricular arrhythmias (T de P*) AVOID COMBINATION	High
	Anti-psychotics – all the phenothiazines, amisulpride, haloperidol, pimozide, sertindole	Increased risk of ventricular arrhythmias (T de P*) AVOID COMBINATION	High
	All beta-blockers	Risk of bradycardia, AV block and myocardial depression	High
	sotalol (also a Class III anti-arrhythmic)	Increased risk of ventricular arrhythmias (T de P*) AVOID COMBINATION	High
	diltiazem and verapamil (the calcium-channel blockers)	Increased risk of bradycardia, AV block and myocardial depression – congestive heart failure	High
	ivabradine (new sinus node depressant)	Increased risk of ventricular arrhythmias (T de P*)	High

*T de P = torsade de pointes, a frequently fatal ventricular arrhythmia (*see* Chapter 5 for further details, including those most susceptible to it and therefore most likely to suffer this most severe drug-induced harm, i.e. women, and those with slow heart rate, myocardial disease, hypothyroidism, older age and electrolyte imbalance).

We have just covered three-quarters of the drugs in Table 4.3, for 11 of them give rise to an increased risk of ventricular arrhythmias (*BNF*, Appendix 1: amiodarone) and the possibility of torsade de pointes in susceptible patients. The reason is obvious – all of these drugs can cause myocardial arrhythmia on their own. Prescribing them for a patient who is already taking amiodarone (or vice versa) increases the risk arithmetically or more.

Sotalol, a non-selective beta-blocker, is also, like amiodarone, a Class III anti-arrhythmic drug. The combination of the two clearly gives rise to a high risk of adverse effect, which is accentuated if hypokalaemia is present.

The other beta-blockers are all myocardial depressants, contraindicated in patients with moderate or severe heart block or with worsening, unstable heart failure. The risks noted in Table 4.3 are only to be expected. Likewise, the two calcium-channel blockers with greatest cardiac impact – diltiazem and verapamil – are likely to cause bradycardia, AV block and myocardial depression if given in conjunction with amiodarone.

Importantly, amiodarone is contraindicated for any patient taking lithium, one of whose side-effects is cardiac arrhythmia.

Ivabradine, a new drug that inhibits the sinu–atrial node, is in its 'special reporting' phase. It carries many contraindications, including its use with amiodarone.

3 Adverse renal interactions between amiodarone and other drugs

TABLE 4.4 Adverse renal interactions

Interactions	Drugs interacting	Nature of risk(s)	Risk level
Renal excretion: *proximal convoluted tubular excretion is inhibited by amiodarone*	lithium	Risk of ventricular arrhythmias AVOID COMBINATION	High
	digoxin	Risk of digoxin toxicity AVOID COMBINATION	High
Other renal drug interactions involving amiodarone	Loop and thiazide diuretics and acetazolamide cause hypokalaemia	1 Increase the risk of amiodarone-induced cardiac toxicity. 2 *All diuretics increase the risk of amiodarone-induced cardiac toxicity*	High if hypokalaemia is present

(*continued*)

Interactions	Drugs interacting	Nature of risk(s)	Risk level
	eplerenone	Increased plasma concentration of eplerenone (*see also* effect of eplerenone on amiodarone; see above)	High if hypokalaemia is present
Mechanism unknown	simvastatin	Increased risk of simvastatin-induced myopathy	

The proximal convoluted tubular cells are equipped with several carrier mechanisms whose function is the unidirectional efflux of polarised molecules including drugs and drug metabolites into the tubular lumen and out of the body. Amiodarone inhibits one of these carriers, the P-glycoprotein (Pgp), thus reducing the excretion of digoxin. The *BNF* recommends the halving of the dose of digoxin whenever amiodarone is co-prescribed. *Amiodarone may also reduce digoxin metabolism in the liver by inhibiting a liver transporter (oatp2).*

The other drug–drug interactions of amiodarone associated with the kidney (*see* Table 4.4) are due to plasma electrolyte imbalances caused by all diuretics used as a maintenance therapy. Hypokalaemia is the main risk factor, increasing the possibility of amiodarone-induced myocardial toxicity. Chapters 6 and 7 will cover these problems in greater detail.

Finally, the last item in Table 4.4, simvastatin – that almost ubiquitous prophylactic and therapeutic imperative! The *BNF*, Appendix 1 (amiodarone) states that co-prescribing of simvastatin and amiodarone increases the risk of simvastatin-induced myopathy. The mechanism is unknown at present.

Truly, amiodarone is one of our riskiest drugs, but armed with the knowledge in this chapter, the careful prescriber can use it safely.

REFERENCES

1 McGavock H. *How Drugs Work*. 2nd ed. Oxford: Radcliffe Publishing; 2005.
2 Joint Formulary Committee. *British National Formulary*. 56th ed. London: British Medical Association and Royal Pharmaceutical Society of Great Britain; 2008.

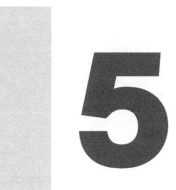

5

The non-steroidal anti-inflammatory drugs (NSAIDs), including the 'COXIB' NSAIDs

If amiodarone is the riskiest drug prescribed in primary care (on specialist recommendation), then the NSAIDs come a close second. Indeed, in epidemiological terms, they are by far the commonest cause of serious drug harm and death reported year on year to government agencies across the world – around 30% of all 'yellow card' reports to the UK's Committee on Safety of Medicines – and the newer 'COXIB' NSAIDs are as frequently reported as the older drugs.

Fortunately, the causes of NSAID-induced adverse drug reactions (ADRs) and adverse drug interactions (ADIs) are relatively easy to explain and understand. NSAIDs block the synthesis within tissue cells of the prostanoid family of chemical messengers – the prostaglandins, prostacyclins and thromboxanes. Several of these are among the chemical messengers that 'trigger' the inflammatory processes. By blocking synthesis of these triggers, the NSAIDs greatly attenuate all inflammation, and are very valuable in managing rheumatoid arthritis and other inflammatory processes, by reducing vasodilatation, oedema and pain. The NSAIDs' analgesic and antipyretic effects are due to blocking of neuronal prostaglandin synthesis, which sensitises peripheral pain receptors and spinal pain pathways, and synthesis of the prostaglandin in the temperature regulator of the hypothalamus, which initiates fever.

However, many non-inflammatory prostanoids are essential chemical messengers that take part in the normal physiological regulation of many tissue and organ functions throughout the body. Unfortunately, the NSAIDs block the synthesis of most of these essential regulators and so seriously disrupt organ function in a large proportion of patients, particularly the elderly and those with failing organs. NSAIDs also interact with several commonly prescribed maintenance regimes, either by reducing their efficacy or by adding to their unwanted side-effects.

The quickest and most dramatic way of revealing the true extent of NSAID harm is to pose a hypothetical clinical scenario: You return from a fortnight's holiday and your first surgery is a nightmare of serious illness, all caused by your deputy's prescribing of an NSAID to patients while you were away (*see* Box 5.1).

BOX 5.1 **What prescribing an NSAID may cause**

1 Bleeding/bruising in a previously well-anticoagulated patient.
2 Acute renal failure in a patient with mild, chronic renal failure.
3 Exacerbation of ulcerative colitis in a previously quiescent case.
4 Acute severe asthma (first attack in 10 years).
5 Flare-up of quiescent psoriasis.
6 Loss of antihypertensive control in a previously stable patient.
7 Worsening of heart failure status in a previously stable elderly man.
8 Flare-up of an old peptic ulcer.
9 Patient previously stable on an ACEI and bendrofluazide is admitted to A & E and found to have severe hyperkalaemia.

You wish that you had not gone on holiday!

Many prescribers are unaware of more than half of these quite common drug-induced events. To remember this catalogue of horrors is essential, but it is also important to understand the mechanisms by which they occur, so

far as they are known. Knowing our drugs' actions – bad as well as good
– is the hallmark of a modern physician (*see* Box 5.2).

BOX 5.2 **Reasons for the serious NSAID-caused events in Box 5.1**

1 The bleeding/bruising was due to the anti-platelet effect of NSAIDs
– they reduce synthesis of the clotting initiator, thromboxane, and
enhance the action of warfarin.

2 In chronic renal failure, the circulation of blood to the renal tubules (via
the efferent arterioles) is dependent on local secretion of prostaglandins
PGI_2 and PGE_2. Three days' use of an NSAID is enough to precipitate
acute renal failure in such patients. Ask your area renal physician.

3 The reason for ulcerative colitis exacerbation is unknown.

4 Most family doctors know that no NSAID (including aspirin) should be
taken by anyone with any history of asthma, however long ago. The
bronchioles are partly dependent on prostaglandin PGE_2 modulation
of smooth muscle tone, to maintain normal patency. If this essential
prostaglandin secretion is blocked by an NSAID, an imbalance of
unopposed broncho-constriction triggers the asthmatic process.

5 The reason for the psoriasis flare-up is not known.

6 NSAIDs significantly antagonise the effect of most anti-hypertensives.
There is an extra risk if NSAIDs are given to patients who are taking
angiotensin-converting-enzyme inhibitors (ACEIs) – an increased risk of
renal impairment and hyperkalaemia (*see also* Chapter 6).

7 NSAIDs should be avoided where possible in any degree of heart failure – they cause increased retention of sodium and water due to a
reduction of renal perfusion. They also have a depressant effect on the
myocardium.

8 Peptic ulceration, the best known of the NSAID ADRs, occurs because
the gastric mucosa is dependent on prostaglandin PGE_2 to inhibit gastric
acid secretion and maintain the protective gastric mucus covering. The
COXIB NSAIDs are less likely to cause peptic ulceration.

9 Anyone prescribing an NSAID to a patient on an ACEI must monitor plasma
electrolytes regularly. Both drug groups indirectly reduce aldosterone
secretion, leading to sodium loss and potassium retention.

FOUR RULES FOR PRESCRIBING NSAIDS

1 If there is no inflammation, give a plain analgesic.
2 Watch like a hawk any patient on long-term NSAIDs – they are only as safe as their prescriber's surveillance.
3 If something unexpected happens, like scenarios 1 to 9 listed above, ask the patient if they have taken an NSAID obtained over the counter or from a relative or neighbour. These dangerous drugs are now licensed for general sale on the shelves of every supermarket and convenience store for analgesia in anyone from toddlers to the elderly. So much for our regulatory watchdogs!
4 Where an NSAID prescription is unavoidable, ibuprofen, naproxen and diclofenac appear to be somewhat less risky than the other NSAIDs.

CONCLUSION

Like warfarin and amiodarone, the NSAIDs are effective but very risky drugs. Their risks are acceptable only in patients whose symptoms and disease progression justify their use.

6

6

Drugs that disrupt the fine equilibrium of renal function

A common A & E 'salvage' operation is the rescue from certain death of patients whose plasma electrolyte balance has been dangerously disrupted by prescribed drugs – every ion may be deficient or excessive in concentration, and the plasma pH and water balance may be upset. Sadly, the 'salvage' operation sometimes fails, and the patient dies due to failure of the prescriber to understand the following relatively simple facts:

1 Revision

Remember that the adrenal hormone, aldosterone, causes sodium ion and water retention and potassium and hydrogen ion excretion by the kidneys. Hence, over-secretion of aldosterone results in excessive Na^+ and water retention, an increase in extracellular fluid volume, hypokalaemia, alkalosis and hypertension. Under-secretion of aldosterone causes net Na^+ loss, water loss, a decrease in extracellular fluid volume, hyperkalaemia and hypotension.

Remember also that aldosterone secretion is stimulated directly by low

Na^+ or high K^+ concentrations in plasma reaching the adrenal gland, and indirectly by a fall in Na^+ concentration in the distal convoluted tubule and/or a fall in the renal arteriolar perfusion pressure. These stimulate the release of renin, which splits-off angiotensin I. Angiotensin-converting enzyme (ACE) converts angiotensin I to angiotensin II (AT II), the potent vasoconstrictor. A further step produces angiotensin III (AT III). Both AT II and AT III stimulate aldosterone secretion, conserving Na^+ and water.

Because three of the six drugs often causing electrolyte imbalance act as partial aldosterone antagonists, this revises all you need as background to understand how everyday prescribing can cause serious electrolyte imbalances, and help you to avoid them. The problem drugs and rationale are set out in Box 6.1. If you doubt the importance of this basic medical science to the family doctor, ask your area A & E consultant how often they are faced with unconscious patients due to one or more of the causes in Box 6.1.

BOX 6.1 **The therapeutic minefield drugs that disrupt the fine equilibrium of renal function, namely spironolactone, the ACEIs and ARBs, the NSAIDs, and the loop and thiazide diuretics**

1 *Spironolactone* and *eplerenone* are aldosterone antagonists. They therefore promote Na^+ loss and K^+ retention.
   (Amiloride and triamterene block inward renal collecting duct Na^+ channels opened by aldosterone, causing Na^+ loss).

2 *Angiotensin-converting-enzyme inhibitors (ACEIs)* and *angiotensin-receptor blockers (ARBs)* block angiotensin II and III synthesis. ATII and ATIII are stimulants for aldosterone release. Hence ACEIs promote Na^+ loss and K^+ retention, by reducing ATII and ATIII levels.

3 *NSAIDs* are indirect renin and aldosterone antagonists – they inhibit renal PGE_2 and PGI_2 synthesis. The result is Na^+ loss and K^+ retention. NSAIDs also reduce renal tubular perfusion by causing constriction of the efferent arterioles.

4 *Loop diuretics* promote K^+ loss and cause Na^+, Mg^{2+} and Ca^{2+} depletion, especially in the elderly.

5 With *thiazides* in low dose, serious side-effects are rare, but K^+ depletion may occur over many months in the elderly. Plasma uric acid levels may also rise.

Here is an actual clinical case submitted by a family doctor colleague.

ACTUAL CLINICAL CASE

1 A doctor and/or nurse has co-prescribed furosemide, an ACEI, an NSAID and spironolactone to a 70-year-old retired labourer. He collapses one week later.
2 The electrolytic result and reason for the collapse.
   - furosemide – loss of K^+, Na^+, Mg^{2+} and Ca^{2+}
   - ACEI – Na^+ loss and K^+ retention
   - NSAID – Na^+ loss and K^+ retention
   - spironolactone – Na^+ loss and K^+ retention
   overall result – profound hyponatraemia and moderate hyperkalaemia, a life-threatening metabolic emergency, which took 48 hours to correct

Ask an A & E consultant how often they have encountered unconscious patients with a similar history. This is happening *now*, somewhere in the UK, every day.

Consider the items in Box 6.1 separately:

1 *Spirolactone* and *eplerenone* are, of course, primarily aldosterone antagonists. They therefore promote Na^+ and water loss and K^+ retention. Their use has increased as 'add-on' therapy in the management of severe congestive heart failure. These are the very patients:
   - who are most likely to have poor renal function
   - whose myocardium is most vulnerable to hyperkalaemia
   - who are often taking digoxin.

2 The *ACEIs* and *ARBs* are among the most useful and frequently used cardiovascular drugs. Not every prescriber realises that they are all indirect aldosterone antagonists, leading to Na^+ loss and K^+ retention. This is because, by definition, ACEIs block the synthesis of ATII and ATIII, both of which stimulate aldosterone release. The ARBs block the angiotensin receptors in the adrenal cortex on which ATII and ATIII act. The result, in either case, is reduced aldosterone secretion. This is rarely a problem in healthy hypertensive patients with normal kidneys,

but patients with any degree of chronic kidney failure require regular plasma electrolyte monitoring. As with spironalactone and thiazide diuretics (see below), the development of clinically significant electrolyte imbalance is usually insidious, and only regular monitoring will give the necessary warning.

An important second factor in ACEI treatment, which is often not understood, is that ACEIs and, to a lesser extent, ARBs reduce the glomerular filtration rate (GFR) by around 20%. This is only a problem if the patient's renal function is reduced, where it complicates the maintenance of water, electrolyte and urea homeostasis and reduces the rate of excretion of many drugs and drug metabolites. Occasionally, ACEIs can cause acute renal failure in patients with chronic renal failure. Here again monitoring is the only safe and scientific way to optimise treatment and minimise its risks.

3   Adverse renal effects of the NSAIDS, old and new.

Chapter 3 explained the risks of NSAIDs to the kidneys. For example, only a few days of NSAID consumption at normal dosage can precipitate acute renal failure in a patient with chronic renal failure. This fact is not as widely understood as it ought to be. Even fewer prescribers know that all NSAIDs are indirect suppressors of renin and aldosterone secretion, resulting in Na^+ and water loss and K^+ retention.

Like the ACEIs, all NSAIDs, including aspirin, reduce renal tubular perfusion, particularly in patients with chronic renal failure. This is because NSAIDs prevent the synthesis of the vasodilator prostaglandin, upon which the efferent renal arterioles depend, in renal failure. The resulting ischaemia of the renal tubules may lead to renal tubular necrosis.

There are two 'take-home' messages:

● Avoid NSAIDs unless inflammation is present, and remember how easily renal function can now be assessed by eGFR and serum creatinine, and consequently how easy it is for the modern family doctor to monitor renal function and diagnose renal failure. Remember, too, that urine dipsticks are very poor predictors of chronic renal failure – microalbuminuria must be sought, and dipsticks will not detect this.

● If the use of NSAIDs in patients with chronic renal failure is unavoidable, maintain a steady clinical concern, monitor their eGFR and electrolytes monthly, and ensure that all your practice colleagues understand the risks – these are 'red flag' patients. A sudden reduction in eGFR (or even in the patient's health) merits immediate admission to the regional renal unit with full clinical referral details.

4 The diuretics – worth watching!

You would expect diuretics to alter the plasma electrolyte balance, because the increased water loss that they cause is secondary to an increased excretion of sodium chloride (NaCl). The greatest risk of serious problems is with the loop diuretics, furosemide and bumetamide, but there is also a risk with long-term, low-dose thiazides.

THE LOOP DIURETICS

These deplete all of the main plasma cations – primarily K^+, but also Na^+, Ca^{2+} and Mg^{2+}. The elderly and patients in chronic renal failure are most at risk, but hypokalaemia, hyponatraemia, hypocalcaemia and hypomagnesaemia can occur at any age and without renal impairment in patients who are taking loop diuretics. The clinical signs of hyponatraemia before collapse and coma supervene are quite unspecific – lethargy, weakness and confusion, easily dismissed in very elderly patients – and the definitive diagnosis can only be made by urgent plasma electrolyte estimation, following the clinician's high index of suspicion. This may pre-empt difficult A & E rescue treatment, which is not always successful. A diagnosis of hyponatraemia is a medical emergency, requiring immediate admission in a fully staffed ambulance.

THE THIAZIDE DIURETICS

These should always be used in low dosage (e.g. bendroflumethiazide 2.5 mg daily), and are usually very safe and effective first-line hypotensive therapy. However, even at low dosage and with healthy kidneys, there is a small relative K^+ depletion from the distal convoluted tubule. If dietary sources of K^+ are persistently inadequate, the plasma K^+ concentration may slowly fall, over many months, and the early symptoms of weakness, fatigue and muscle cramps are easily overlooked. A further decrease in K^+ concentration may present as flaccid paralysis and will result in emergency admission to A & E, where electrolyte estimation and ECG will confirm the diagnosis. Particularly at risk are patients taking digoxin, since hypokalaemia increases the risk of digitalis toxicity. Therefore patients who are taking low-dose thiazides should also be regularly monitored, every six months for those least at risk, and every three months for those most at risk, not forgetting those who are unable to attend the medical centre (the district nurse will gladly take blood for electrolyte estimation).

CONCLUSION

Armed with the information in this chapter, the informed prescriber will have no difficulty in avoiding the common pitfalls listed in Box 6.1. The messages are threefold:

1 Monitor the plasma electrolytes and eGFR regularly in all patients who are taking the drugs listed in Box 6.1, *particularly any combination of them*. It takes about two minutes to do this, but can save lives. Don't forget housebound patients.

2 Remember that those at greatest risk are patients with reduced eGFR, particularly the elderly.

3 Warn all patients who are taking the drugs in Box 6.1 not to buy any painkillers in any shop, even a pharmacy – and to use only analgesics prescribed by you. (And restrict your own use of NSAIDs for such patients to unavoidable cases).

7

7

Sudden cardiac collapse due to often-prescribed drugs causing QT$_c$ prolongation

As all clinicians know, the conventional ECG wave points are identified as PQRST, from P, the atrial contraction, to T, the ventricular repolarisation wave. The length of the ventricular section, from Q to the end of T, is the QT interval. For comparison of different patients, each individual's QT length in milliseconds is converted (or standardised) to what it would have been if their heart rate had been 60 beats/minute. This approximation is the QT corrected (or QT$_c$) interval.

If the QT$_c$ interval is much prolonged, the ventricular contraction sequence is severely disrupted, leading to a characteristic ECG trace of 'atypical' ventricular dysrhythmia called 'torsade de pointes' (twisted points). Figure 7.1 shows the onset of this fearful event. As you can see, the QRS trace 'twists around' the ECG baseline. Syncope is immediate, and collapse and death often follow rapidly, if the patient is not under the care of a cardiologist or A & E physician with the requisite knowledge, skills and drugs.

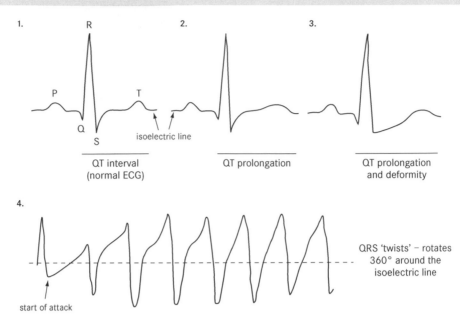

FIGURE 7.1 ECG of Torsade de Pointes (polymorphic ventricular tachycardia)

The commonest cause of torsade de pointes appears to be the prescription of certain drugs to patients who are predisposed to the condition. Box 7.1 lists the known risk factors for drug-induced torsade de pointes. The use of practice computers makes it possible to conduct a search for a convergence of two or more of these known risk factors, which would signal the need for caution in prescribing any of the drugs/drug groups in Box 7.2, for it indicates a 5- to 10-fold increased risk. Three or more risk factors incur a progressively greater risk. Where the use of a drug listed in Box 7.2 is unavoidable, it is certainly advisable to share the prescribing decision with a specialist colleague. The use of two drugs listed in Box 7.2 increases the risk of torsade de pointes to an even greater degree, and the expected benefit would have to exceed this risk substantially before it could be justified.

BOX 7.1 Known risk factors for drug-induced torsade de pointes

1 Female sex
2 A genetic variant for cardiac ion transport
3 Any pre-existing myocardial disease, including recent atrial fibrillation
4 Increasing age
5 Hypothyroidisn
6 Bradycardia
7 Hypokalaemia
8 Hypomagnesaemia
9 Pre-existing QT prolongation (usually due to 1 and 2 above).

BOX 7.2 Commonly used drugs that prolong the QT_c interval, risking torsade de pointes ventricular arrhythmia

1 **Cardiac drugs**
    amiodarone
    sotalol
    disopyramide
    procainamide
2 **Antibacterials**
    erythromycin
    clarithromycin
    moxifloxacin
    pentamidine
3 **Calcium-channel blockers**
    diltiazem
    verapamil
4 **Antipsychotics**
    All of the older (phenothiazine) drugs
    haloperidol
    pimozide
    sertindole
    amisulpride

5 **Antidepressants**
All tricyclics, particularly dosulepin (Prothiaden)
fluvoxamine
paroxetine
lithium

6 **Anti-emetics**
domperidone

7 **Anti-fungals**
ketoconazole

8 **Antihistamines**
mizolastine

9 **Analgesics**
methadone

The risk of serious arrhythmia in the general population is probably 1% or lower, but rises significantly in predisposed patients (see above) *and* if two or more of these drugs are co-prescribed. As with all prescribing risks, knowledge is strength!

8

INTRODUCTION TO CHAPTERS 8 AND 9: DRUG INTERACTIONS

Drugs interact with other drugs in two quite distinct ways, both of which have important implications for the prescriber and potentially serious ones for the patient.

1 Chapter 8 discusses drugs interacting at their shared sites of action and/or therapeutic effect – the so-called 'pharmacodynamic' interactions.

2 Chapter 9 discusses the complex nature of adverse drug–drug interactions during drug metabolism in the liver. This is one of the commonest and most serious causes of unintentional but preventable prescription-related disease (PPRD). The jargon for it is 'pharmacokinetic' drug interaction.

8

Some important interactions between drugs at shared sites of action and/or therapeutic effect

An excellent way of grasping this basic concept is to remember how often we co-prescribe two or more potent drugs to in order to 'normalise' pathophysiology. Everyday examples include the following:

1 Refractory hypertension often needs a combination of an ACEI, a calcium-channel blocker, a diuretic and an alpha-blocker to achieve adequate control. All of these act in different ways to reduce peripheral resistance (verapamil and diltiazem also depress the myocardium), and together in moderate dosage may achieve better control than one or two drugs in high dosage (see *Treating Common Diseases*, Chapter 1).[1]

2 Severe rheumatoid arthritis is a lifelong destructive disease that requires early diagnosis and treatment to avoid the joint erosion which begins within a few months of onset (see *Treating Common Diseases*, Chapter 12).[1] An NSAID is virtually an automatic first choice, often followed by a weekly oral dose of methotrexate, which reduces the immune response, with the option of adding one or more further disease-modifying anti-rheumatic drugs (DMARDs) like etanercept or

infliximab, which inhibit cytokines (chemical messengers which drive part of the inflammatory process). All of these agents act to reduce inflammation in the tissues, and may be used synergistically in lower and therefore less toxic doses than in monotherapy, thus achieving better disease control with fewer side-effects.

3 Cancer chemotherapy today usually involves the use of two or more anti-metabolites, often combined with high-dose steroids and anti-emetics to counter their severe side-effects.

4 HIV infection now requires three antiviral drugs (*see BNF*). Each drug acts to disrupt a different element of retroviral metabolism. The virus may have developed resistance to any two of these drugs, but rarely to all three.

Doctors are well aware of such synergistic prescribing, which includes the treatment of asthma, type 2 diabetes and hyperlipidaemia. Practice has shown them that most of these combinations 'balance' quite well, with tolerable side-effects in the long term. Problems tend to occur when another drug is added. It is worth revising several important adverse drug interactions in treatment regimens for cardiovascular disease, asthma and the specialist-led treatment of depression and psychosis.

HYPERTENSION AND CONGESTIVE HEART FAILURE

As Chapter 3 showed, in regimens for hypertension and congestive heart failure (CHF), NSAIDs will cause significant deterioration of control. There is a particular risk in prescribing an NSAID (or the patient taking an OTC NSAID) for any patient on an ACEI or ARB, as both drugs reduce renal function by around 20% and both cause hyperkalaemia. NSAIDs should be avoided, or a different hypotensive chosen. In addition, any NSAID will reduce the hypotensive effect of any antihypertensive regimen through loading of extra Na^+ and water, made worse by blocking the positive inotropic effect of physiological prostaglandins on the myocardium.

Although it is now common for cardiologists to advise the use of low-dose beta-blockers like bisoprolol or carvedilol as 'add-on' therapy in severe CHF, the family doctor, as the physician in overall charge, needs to watch for a worsening of the CHF due to the negative inotropic effect of the beta-blockers, reducing cardiac contractility. Do not hesitate to stop the beta-blocker if symptoms and signs indicate deterioration.

ERECTION ENHANCERS

A 'wonder-drug' group now widely available without prescription are the erection enhancers – sildenafil, tadalafil and vardenafil. These pose a great risk to all patients taking slow-release nitrates for angina. Their potent vasodilation is not confined to the penis, and can cause widespread systemic vasodilation, profound hypotension and collapse in a patient who is taking a slow-release nitrate. Since the nitrate is usually long-acting or sustained release, the long-acting tadalafil and vardenafil carry a greater risk in such a drug–drug interaction. A paramedic ambulance and immediate A & E admission are essential, for rescue is not always successful.

As Chapter 2 showed, men who are using an erection enhancer should not take grapefruit juice, grapefruit or bitter oranges, as they increase the bioavailability of the erection enhancers.

This is a sensible point at which to remind all prescribers of the contraindications to erection enhancers:
1 Do not use in hypotensive patients.
2 Do not use after a recent stroke.
3 Do not use within six months of a myocardial infarction.
4 Do not use in unstable angina.
5 Take extra care when prescribing for patients with multiple myeloma or leukaemia.
6 Examine the penis for anatomical abnormality before prescribing.

The author suggests a further warning: tell all angina patients who are taking slow-release nitrates to avoid erection enhancers, and record your warning in the patient's records.

CARDIAC ARRHYTHMIAS

The main interaction risk of all anti-arrhythmic drugs with other drugs is a synergistic depression of both the cardiac conducting tissues and the general myocardium. There is, of course, a major risk if two anti-arrhythmic drugs are co-prescribed. The other major risk is prescribing an anti-arrhythmic drug to any patient who is taking digoxin.

1 Amiodarone added to digoxin incurs a high risk of acute heart failure and asystole (*see* Chapter 4).
2 The most powerful calcium-channel blockers – diltiazem and verapamil – may precipitate CHF if ventricular function is borderline.

Such drug combinations are best used only on specialist recommendation after echocardiogram assessment and with regular plasma electrolyte monitoring.

ADVERSE DRUG INTERACTIONS IN THE LUNGS

Because of their frequency of prescribing and OTC availability, NSAIDs pose the greatest risk for asthmatic patients. Not only may NSAIDs, including aspirin, precipitate wheeze and often acute severe asthma in any asthmatic, but also in an asthmatic patient who is well controlled by steroid inhalations, they will adversely affect the quality of control, even if they do not cause frank symptoms.

The other main risk for asthmatic patients is the use of any beta-blocker, including bisoprolol, carvedilol and even timolol eye drops. Not only is such use likely to cause severe acute asthma, but because of a drug interaction, rescue of the patient may be very difficult. Although bisoprolol and carvedilol are described as 'selective' for β_1-receptors, this selectivity is only relative, and there is always some blockade of the bronchodilator β_2-adrenergic receptors in the airways. That means that the effect of the bronchodilators salbutamol and terbutaline is much reduced – the β_2-receptors in bronchial smooth muscle are blocked and unresponsive to the β_2-agonists – a major A & E emergency.

A separate topic – drug-induced lung disease – is covered in Chapter 12.

ADVERSE DRUG INTERACTIONS IN THE CENTRAL NERVOUS SYSTEM (CNS)

Mental and neurological illness may strike at almost any age and in any state of health, and drug treatment is obligatory for moderate and severe depression, all psychoses and many neurological syndromes, irrespective of whether the patient is otherwise well, taking no medicine, or having multiple drug treatment for a somatic disease. The interaction between CNS drugs and many somatic regimens is a vast and complex topic. To 'short-circuit' some of this complexity, and awaken readers to the problems, please open your most recent *BNF* and spend an hour studying the cautions and side-effects for the tricyclic (TCA) and selective serotonin reuptake inhibitor (SSRI) antidepressants, the new and older antipsychotics and lithium, and the anti-epileptics in the main body of the *BNF*.[2] Then study the known important drug–drug interactions of these same therapies, in Appendix 1 of the *BNF*. You will find your study both interesting and worrying!

Psychiatrists and neurologists are accustomed to creating effective and tolerable treatment regimens and to making allowance for essential co-prescribing of drugs for somatic illness. This makes it especially important for the family doctor, in a referral letter, to inform the specialist of every detail of the patient's somatic diagnoses and drug treatment. Likewise, in a psychiatric or neurological patient who is stabilised on therapy, all of the practice team must realise the importance of consulting the psychiatrist or neurologist *before adding any new drug treatment*. Ask your area specialists how often this is not done, and what chaos results!

REFERENCES

1 McGavock H and Johnston D. *Treating Common Diseases*. Oxford: Radcliffe Publishing; 2007.
2 Joint Formulary Committee. *British National Formulary*. 56th ed. London: British Medical Association and Royal Pharmaceutical Society of Great Britain; 2008.

9

Major prescribing pitfalls due to drug–drug interactions in the liver

No drug is suitable for prescribing unless it can be inactivated by metabolism, usually in the liver, and/or excreted, usually by the kidneys. The liver has a powerful battery of iso-enzymes, similar in structure and function but each specific only for the metabolism (bioconversion/transformation) of a particular group of drugs or poisons (*see How Drugs Work*, Chapters 3 and 23).[1] This is 'Phase I' metabolism. There are few chemical compounds which cannot be metabolised by this cytochrome P_{450} (CYP_{450}) oxidase capacity, which must have conferred a great evolutionary advantage – it can be found in quite 'primitive' life forms. Other liver enzymes, the conjugation processes, are separate, acting either on individual drugs or on the products of P_{450} metabolites. That is 'Phase II' metabolism.

The problem for the prescriber is that many effective and commonly used drugs interfere with the function of one or more of these P_{450} liver enzymes in one of two ways. Some drugs inhibit P_{450} enzymes, reducing their metabolic effectiveness, while others induce (or stimulate) them, increasing their drug-metabolising function.

ENZYME INHIBITION

If one drug inhibits a liver enzyme which is essential for the metabolism of other drugs, the plasma concentration of those drugs will increase and may reach toxic levels. About 13 drugs/drug groups are potent liver enzyme inhibitors and cause an excessive plasma concentration of scores of other essential drugs whose metabolism is reduced. This is the process which is a major cause of preventable prescription-related disease. Table 9.1 lists the 13 major liver enzyme inhibitors that you need to remember. Box 9.1 is in the form of a sonnet (doggerel) to help you to remember them – you remember 30% of what you hear, 30% of what you read and 30% of what you see, but 100% of every poem that you learn! The right-hand column of Table 9.2 shows you how many important drugs have their metabolism reduced. Do not try to learn these – learn the inhibiting drugs (left-hand column of Table 9.2 and sonnet). Whenever you wish to add one of the 'left-hand' drugs to a patient's regimen, use your computer software to screen for serious interactions with the existing drugs. Conversely, when a patient is taking one of the 'left-hand' drugs regularly, check the drug interaction software before adding another drug. Alternatively, phone your regional Medicines Information Service (see inside front cover of the *BNF* for the phone number and *see* Box 9.2).[2]

TABLE 9.1 Frequently-used drugs which inhibit metabolic enzymes

---

The following drugs *increase the plasma concentration* of other drugs whose metabolism is inhibited, leading to potential toxicity:

- all imidazole antifungals – watch for the suffix '-azole' – affect many other drugs (*see BNF*, Appendix 1)

- cimetidine (Tagamet) – available over the counter, and increases the plasma concentration of over 70 other drugs. One of the very few drugs that inhibit almost all CYP groups; it is available without prescription in the UK

- grapefruit juice (*see* Chapter 2) increases the plasma concentration of over 40 other drugs. Tell patients on maintenance regimes not to drink grapefruit juice or eat grapefruit. A 250-ml glassful knocks out a generation of P_{450} in the intestinal wall – and it takes 24 hours to recover. More than 500 ml/day also knocks out liver CYP 3A4

- macrolides (erythromycin, etc.) – increase the plasma concentration of over 25 other drugs

---

(*continued*)

The following drugs *increase the plasma concentration* of other drugs whose metabolism is inhibited, leading to potential toxicity:

- SSRIs – increase the plasma concentration of over 20 other drugs, including tricyclic antidepressants (TCIs), benzodiazepines and many antipsychotics
- calcium-channel blockers – verapamil and diltiazem – increase the plasma concentration of 14 other drugs
- amiodarone – increases the plasma concentration of 10 other drugs, including warfarin, digoxin and ciclosporin
- metronidazole – increases the plasma concentration of 5 other drugs, including lithium and alcohol
- 4-quinolones (ciprofloxacin, etc.) – increase the plasma concentration of methotrexate and theophylline
- omeprazole (Losec) – increases the plasma concentration of diazepam and digoxin
- allopurinol – increases the plasma concentration of ciclosporin
- sulphonamides – increase the plasma concentration of phenytoin
- antivirals – several of these are enzyme inhibitors, and several are enzyme inducers. (The *BNF* advises consulting Appendix 1 under the individual antiviral drug name.)

See Table 9.2 for further detail showing commonly-used drugs whose metabolism is impaired

---

BOX 9.1 **An interaction elegy or cytochrome sonnet**

- Watch Tagamet and grapefruit juice, azoles and macrolides
- They increase the concentration of many other drugs besides
- So do SSRIs, diltiazem, verapamil and amiodarone
- Metronidazole, omeprazole and the 4-quinolones
- Use EMIS and TOREX software or a pharmacist on the phone
- Allopurinol increases the concentration of ciclosporin
- And sulphonamides do the same for our old friend phenytoin
- Some antivirals inhibit enzymes, others enzymes do induce
- And for these the *BNF*, Appendix 1, you then should use!
- When any of these prescriptions flow from printer or from pen
- Then check for interactions with the patient's drug regimen.

BOX 9.2 **Regional Medicines Information Service phone numbers**

England
Birmingham	+ 44 (0121) 311 1974
Bristol	+44 (0117) 928 2867
Ipswich	+44 (01473) 704 431
Leeds	+44 (0113) 3923547
Leicester	+44 (0116) 255 5779
Liverpool	+44 (0151) 794 8113/4/5/7
	+44 (0151) 794 8206

London
Guy's Hospital	+44 (020) 7188 8750
	+44 (020) 7188 3849
	+44 (020) 7188 3855
Northwick Park Hospital	+44 (020) 8869 3973
	+44 (020) 8869 2763

Newcastle	+44 (0191) 260 6198
Southampton	+44 (023) 8079 6908/9

Wales
Cardiff	+44 (029) 2074 2979
	+44 (029) 2074 2251

Scotland
Aberdeen	+44 (01224) 552 316
Dundee	+44 (01382) 632 351
	+44 (01382) 660 111 ext 32351
Edinburgh	+44 (0131) 242 2920
Glasgow	+44 (0141) 211 4407

Northern Ireland
Belfast	+44 (028) 9063 2032
	+44 (028) 9063 3847

Republic of Ireland
Dublin	Dublin 473 0589
	Dublin 453 7941 ext 2348

TABLE 9.2 Some metabolic enzyme inhibitors frequently used in primary care: these *increase the effect* of drugs where metabolism is inhibited

P450 enzyme inhibitor	Drugs whose plasma concentration is increased
imidazole antifungals, e.g. fluconazole, itraconazole, ketoconazole, etc.	acenocoumarol (nicoumalone), alfentanil, antivirals, ciclosporin, corticosteroids, digoxin, felodipine, midazolam, phenytoin, quinidine, rifabutin, sildenafil, etc., sulphonylureas, tacrolimus, theophylline, warfarin, atypical antipsychotics, terfenadine, calcium-channel blockers, triptans, cilostazol, new anti-malarials
cimetidine 1. avoid this drug, but – 2. it remains available from pharmacies, without prescription: ask patients whether they are taking it	• antihelmintics • anti-arrythmics; amiodarone, flecainide, lidocaine (lignocaine), procainamide, propafenone, quinidine • antibacterials: erythromycin, metronidazole • anticoagulants: acenocoumarol, warfarin • antidepressants: amitriptyline, doxepin, moclobemide, nortriptyline • anti-epileptics: carbamazepine, phenytoin, valproate • antifungals: terbinafine • antihistamines: loratadine • antimalarials: chloroquine, quinine • anxiolytics and hypnotics: benzodiazepines, clomethiazole • beta-blockers: labetalol, propranolol • calcium-channel blockers: some • cytotoxics: fluorouracil • immunosuppressant: ciclosporin (possibly) • NSAIDs: azapropazone (possibly) • opioid analgesics: pethidine • theophylline
omeprazole	diazepam, digoxin (possibly)
lansoprazole	cilostazol (new peripheral vasodilator), clarithromycin, phenytoin, methotrexate, tacrolimus
allupurinol	ciclosporin
erythromycin and other macrolides	alfentanil, amiodarone, bromocriptine, cabergoline, carbamazepine, ciclosporin, clozapine, disopyramide, felodipine, midazolam, rifabutin, sildenafil, theophylline, zopiclone, moxifloxacin, repaglinide, itraconazole, mizolastine, loratadine, atypical antipsychotics, buspirone, zopiclone, digoxin, some statins
ciprofloxacin, norfloxacin	theophylline, methotexate
sulphonamides	phenytoin
amiodarone	acenocoumarol, ciclosporin, digoxin, flecainide, phenytoin, procainamide, quinidine, warfarin

(continued)

P450 enzyme inhibitor	Drugs whose plasma concentration is increased
metronidazole	phenytoin, fluorouracil, primidone, lithium or alcohol
SSRIs	benzodiazepines (some), carbamazepine, clozapine, flecainide, haloperidol, phenytoin, propranolol, theophylline, tricyclic, antidepressants, ropivacaine, NSAIDs, methadone, many antipsychotics
calcium-channel blockers – verapamil, diltiazem	alcohol, ciclosporin, digoxin, imipramine, midazolam, nifedipine, phenytoin, quinidine, theophylline, buspirone, cilostazol, dutasteride, siriolimus
several antivirals: indinavir, ritonavir, nelfinavir, saquinavir (*see BNF*, Appendix 1, under individual drugs for comprehensive list)	erection enhancers (sildenafil, vardenafil, tadalafil), many common analgesics (all NSAIDs, morphine, diamorphine, fentanyl, pethidine, dextropropoxyphene), anti-arrhythmics (amiodarone, flecainide, quinidine, disopyramide, mexiletine, propafenone), macrolide antibiotics (erythromycin, azithromycin, clarithromycin), the SSRI and tricyclic antidepressants, the azole antifungals (itraconazole, ketoconazole), most antipsychotics, most benzodiazepine sedatives, terfenadine, tolterodine, the lipid regulators (atorvastatin, simvastatin)
grapefruit juice and fresh grapefruit. (Most patients on long-term medication should avoid these, as a precaution	calcium-channel blockers (nifedipine, felodipine, verapamil, etc.), erection enhancers (as above), anti-rejection immunosuppressants (ciclosporin, siriolimus, tacrolimus), simvastatin, buspirone, terfenadine, efavirenz, saquinavir, atorvastatin, amiodarone, astemizole, carbamazepine, midazolam, sertraline, triazolam, warfarin
ethyl alcohol	enhances the effect of many drugs (not necessarily via P450 inhibition). See full page in *BNF*, Appendix 1 – you will be amazed and enlightened!

ENZYME INDUCTION

Table 9.3 shows the main drugs that *induce* P_{450} liver enzymes (left-hand column) and the most important drugs whose metabolism is thereby increased, causing a reduction in their plasma concentration. The risk here is clearly not of toxicity, but of *treatment failure*, and a brief study of the right-hand column of Table 9.3 will show just how seriously this could affect a patient. Again, learn only the nine liver enzyme inducers – an easy task – the four anti-epileptics, the rifamycins, St John's wort, griseofulvin and two antivirals. Then use computer screening for interaction with any other drug that you plan to co-prescribe.

A major risk of failing to understand enzyme induction is that the prescriber may attribute treatment failure to an inadequate dose, and increase the dose of the (right-hand column) drug to compensate. If the inducing (left-hand column) drug is then withdrawn, the new dose will be excessive, and will lead to toxicity.

TABLE 9.3 Metabolic enzyme inducers: these *reduce the effect of* drugs whose metabolism is accelerated.

P450 enzyme inducer	Drugs whose plasma concentration is reduced
barbiturates and primidone*	acenocoumarol, amprenavir, atovaquone, benzodiazepines, bisoprolol, carbamazepine, chloramphenicol, chlorpropamide, ciclosporin, cimetidine, corticosteroids, dapsone, digitoxin, diltiazem, disopyramide, fluconazole, fluvastatin, haloperidol, indinavir, itraconazole, ketoconazole, levothyroxine, methadone, mexiletine, nelfinavir, nifedipine, oral contraceptives, phenytoin, propafenone, propranolol, quinidine, simvastatin, siriolimus, tacrolimus, terbinafine, theophylline, tolbutamide, tricyclic antidepressants, verapamil, warfarin
phenytoin*	acenocoumarol (nicoumalone), chloramphenicol, ciclosporin, corticosteroids, digitoxin, disopyramide, doxycycline, gestrinone, indinavir, lamotrigine, levothyroxine (thyroxine), metronidazole, mianserin, oral contraceptives, quinidine, theophylline, tibolone, toremifene, tricyclics, warfarin
carbamazepine*	acenocoumarol, ciclosporin, clozapine, corticosteroids, digitoxin, disopyramide, indinavir, itraconazole, ketoconazole, lamotrigine, methadone, mexiletine, mianserin, oral contraceptives, paroxetine, quetiapine, quinidine, theophylline, thyroxine, warfarin
rifamycins	acenocoumarol, antiepileptics, ciclosporin, corticosteroids, digitoxin, gestrinone, haloperidol, indinavir, mianserin, olanzapine, oral contraceptives, risperidone, theophylline, tibolone, toremifene, tricyclic antidepressants, warfarin
Two antivirals: efavirenz	methadone, rifabutin, sertraline, other antivirals (*see BNF*), oestrogens (risking contraceptive failure)
nevirapine	methadone, warfarin, ketoconazole, other antivirals (*see BNF*), oestrogens and progestogens (risk of contraceptive failure)

(continued)

P450 enzyme inducer	Drugs whose plasma concentration is reduced
St John's Wort – a very common self-medication herbal. Advise all patients on long-term treatment not to use it	many antivirals, telithromycin, warfarin, amitriptyline, carbamazepine, phenytoin, primidone, phenobarbitone, digoxin, simvastatin, theophylline, tacrolimus, cidosporin, oestrogens and progestogens (risk of contraceptive failure)
griseofulvin	acenocoumarol, ciclosporin, oral contraceptives, warfarin

*Combination therapy with two or more anti-epileptic drugs enhances toxicity, and drug interactions may occur between anti-epileptics (*see BNF* Appendix 1, anti-epileptics).

REFERENCES

1 McGavock H. *How Drugs Work*. 2nd ed. Oxford: Radcliffe Publishing; 2005.
2 Joint Formulary Committee. *British National Formulary*. 56th ed. London: British Medical Association and Royal Pharmaceutical Society of Great Britain; 2008.

10

10

Two serious prescribing pitfalls caused by alcohol use (and abuse)

A previous generation, when offering one a drink, often asked 'What's your poison?'! They were much more scientific than they knew, for alcohol is a potent hepatocellular poison and, even in moderate amounts, it disrupts liver function temporarily. The majority of western populations drink alcohol – some occasionally, some regularly and moderately, and some excessively. That truism is important for the prescriber, because alcohol has paradoxical effects on P_{450} liver enzymes which metabolise other drugs (*see* Chapter 9), dependent on the person's drinking habits.

1 *Occasional drinking* inhibits members of the P_{450} enzyme group, reducing the metabolism of many drugs and leading to an increase in their plasma concentration (*see* Chapter 9). The *BNF* (Appendix 1) has two columns citing drugs whose plasma concentration and therapeutic effects are enhanced by the concurrent occasional use of alcohol.[1]

2 Conversely, chronic, regular heavy drinking *induces the same enzymes*, increasing drug metabolism and leading to a reduced plasma drug concentration and therapeutic failure. Singularly, the *BNF* does not

describe this reverse effect of alcohol in chronic drinkers and alcoholics. In these patients, there is a high risk of therapeutic failure in patients who are taking the following drugs/drug groups:

- warfarin
- tolbutamide
- doxycycline
- antidepressants
- antipsychotics
- the benzodiazepines
- paracetamol.

In particular, beware paracetamol overdose in chronic drinkers. Because of enzyme induction, their livers produce more of the toxic paracetamol metabolite N-acetyl-p-benzoquinone imine (NAPBQI), which is the common cause of death in paracetamol poisoning. Alcoholics and heavy drinkers should be warned to avoid paracetamol.

Alcohol itself is metabolised stepwise by two enzymes, alcohol dehydrogenase and aldehyde dehydrogenase, and to a lesser extent by a P_{450} enzyme. Unfortunately, the availability of these enzymes for alcohol is limited, and the metabolic capacity is saturated after only a few drinks. The remaining alcohol after a 'night out' is slowly metabolised over the next 12 hours or more – hence the drink-driving convictions the 'morning after.'

ANTABUSE-LIKE REACTIONS

Most prescribers know that the alcohol aversion drug, disulfiram (Antabuse), causes a progressive series of very unpleasant symptoms, depending on the dose of alcohol consumed. These include vomiting, flushing, headache, palpitations and (if the alcohol intake is large), hypotension and collapse (see the contraindications to disulfiram prescribing in the *BNF*, Chapter 4.10).

However, many prescribers are unaware that a number of commonly prescribed drugs may cause a similar reaction. These are:

- cephalosporins
- metronidazole
- sulfonamides

- isoniazid
- griseofulvin
- sulphonylureas
- nitrofurantoin
- nitrates.

As with disulfiram, the severity of the reaction between these drugs and alcohol is proportional to the dose of alcohol and, at worst, collapse, convulsions and death may result.

REFERENCE

1 Joint Formulary Committee. *British National Formulary.* 56th ed. London: British Medical Association and Royal Pharmaceutical Society of Great Britain; 2008.

11

11

Monitoring the effects of drug treatment to avoid pitfalls. Which drugs? Which tests? How often?

Given the power and risks of modern drugs, clinicians in primary care have come to regard monitoring as a routine part of clinical observation at every review consultation. It becomes so routine that we often forget we are monitoring. Experience leads to increased expectation of the unexpected!

This short chapter presents the main drugs that require watchful, regular monitoring, in an accessible tabular format (*see* Table 11.1), the essential laboratory addition to our clinical observation of expected and unexpected changes resulting from drug treatment. The author is indebted to colleagues at the Northern Ireland Regional Medicines and Poisons Information Service, for permission to publish Table 11.1 from their drug information bulletin *Drug Data*, Volume 46, originally published in 1998. Readers may consider giving a copy to all family doctor colleagues and organising a seminar on drug monitoring for treatment room nurses, who are often responsible for carrying out venesection for these tests – they have been shown to be rather better at following protocols than many doctors!

TABLE 11.1 Monitoring for adverse effects of drug treatment

Drug	Tests before therapy	Serum drug levels		Tests during therapy	Frequency	Notes
		Range	Frequency			
ACE inhibitors	Urea, creatinine, renal function, electrolytes			Urea, creatinine, electrolytes	14 days after starting treatment and then periodically	
Amiodarone	Thyroid function, chest X-ray, liver function			Thyroid function, liver function	Every 6 months	If pulmonary toxicity suspected, chest X-ray and lung function tests
Azathioprine				Full blood picture, differential white cell count	Weekly for first 8 weeks then monthly	
Carbimazole Propylthiouracil				White cell count Free thyroxine levels	Within 3 months of starting treatment Every 4–6 weeks until hyperthyroidism controlled then 3–6 monthly	Patient warned to report sore throat immediately (risk of agranulocytosis with carbimazole)
Clozapine	Full blood picture, differential white cell count			Full blood picture, differential white cell count	Weekly for first 18 weeks then every 2 weeks for 1 year then monthly	Monitoring carried out by Clozaril Patient Monitoring Service

Drug	Tests before therapy	Serum drug levels		Tests during therapy	Frequency	Notes
		Range	Frequency			
Cyclophosphamide				Full blood picture, differential white cell count, urinalysis	Weekly for first 8 weeks then monthly	
Ciclosporin	Blood pressure, serum creatinine, urea, bilirubin, liver enzymes, blood lipids	Trough varies according to indication	Varies according to indication	Serum creatinine, urea, potassium, bilirubin, liver enzymes, blood lipids, blood pressure	Weekly initially then every 4 weeks	Check trough level if adding or stopping drug known to affect ciclosporine levels. Avoid high dietary potassium
Digoxin	Kidney function, potassium, thyroid function	> 2 microgram/l increased risk of toxicity	Day 7, then periodically	Kidney function, potassium, thyroid function	Periodically	Repeat level 1 week after adding or stopping any interacting drug
Diuretics NB thiazides as well as loop diuretics				Serum electrolytes and eGFR	Periodically	Repeat tests after adding or removing any interacting drug
Erythropoietin	Haemoglobin, iron status, faecal occult blood, Coomb's test, blood pressure			Full blood picture, iron status	Monthly	
				Blood pressure	Weekly	

(continued)

Drug	Tests before therapy	Serum drug levels		Tests during therapy	Frequency	Notes
		Range	Frequency			
Gold	No			Full blood picture, differential white cell count, urinalysis	Intramuscular – before each injection Oral – monthly	
Lithium		0.4–1.0 mmol/l	After 4–7 days, then weekly until constant for 4 weeks, then every 3 months	Thyroid function	Initially every 6 months then annually	Measure drug level 12 hours after dose
Methotrexate	Renal and liver function, full blood count, proteinuria, haematuria			Full blood picture, differential white cell count, renal and liver function tests	Fortnightly for first 3 months then monthly	Patient asked to report immediately any sore throat or other infection.
Penicillamine				Full blood picture, differential white cell count, urinalysis	Fortnightly for firs 6 weeks then monthly	Repeat tests one week after any dose increase. 'See Cautions *BNF*'
Statins	Liver function			Liver enzymes, creatine kinase	First 4 months and then periodically	

Drug	Tests before therapy	Serum drug levels		Tests during therapy	Frequency	Notes
		Range	Frequency			
Sulphasalazine	Full blood picture, differential white cell count			Full blood picture, differential white cell count Liver function	Monthly for first 3 months then every 6 months Monthly for first 3 months	Abnormalities usually occur within the first 3–6 months and are reversible on stopping
Vitamin D	No			Serum calcium Serum creatinine if receiving calcitriol	Initially weekly At 4 weeks, 3 and 6 months and then 6-monthly	Where pharmacological doses are prescribed
Warfarin	No			INR	Daily or on alternate days initially, then at longer intervals (depending on response) then up to every 8 weeks	Repeat INR one week after adding or stopping an interacting drug

Reproduced from Drug Data, 46; 1998, updated with permission from Professor GPR Archbold, Consultant in Clinical Biochemistry, Belfast City Hospital.

The great strength of Table 11.1 is that it specifies:
1 pre-treatment tests to establish a baseline
2 the desirable therapeutic range (where appropriate)
3 the frequency of test repetition for therapeutic range
4 tests during maintenance therapy to detect known adverse effects of the drug regimens
5 the frequency of test repetition
6 further special monitoring.

No further explanation is needed for the established family doctor.

Please note the increasing use of the disease modifying anti-rheumatic drugs (DMARDs), methotrexate, azathioprine, ciclosporin, cyclophosphamide and leflunomide has extended the need for monitoring adverse effects, particularly on the haemopoietic system. These drugs are almost always consultant-initiated and GPs should seek precise follow-up protocols from the consultant concerned. The same applies to the even more toxic cytokine modulators adalimumab, anakinra, etanercept and infliximab. *BNF* Chapter 10.1.3 devotes six pages to the use of and problems associated with these new, effective but very risky drugs. Above all, no changes should be made in a patient's drug regimen without reference to the consultant in charge.

12

12

Serious lung diseases caused by prescribed drugs

It is impossible for any doctor to know too much, particularly the general practitioner! This is because less common diagnoses will only be made if the doctor knows of them and has considered them when 'scanning' the differential diagnoses, as we all do, consciously or unconsciously, when faced with a patient whose symptoms and clinical findings do not indicate one of the commoner conditions.

Nowhere is this dictum more important than in the lungs. The common lung diseases are few in number and mostly easily diagnosed – asthma, bronchitis, chronic obstructive pulmonary disease (COPD), pneumonia, pleurisy, tuberculosis, pleural effusion (from whatever cause) and cancers. Likewise, most doctors are well aware of the serious risks of prescribing beta-blockers (even eye drops) or any NSAID to any patient with a history of asthma, and the chronic dry cough that ACEIs cause in a small proportion of patients.

Many commonly used drugs, mainly medicinal but including drugs of abuse (heroin, cocaine and crack cocaine) occasionally cause serious lung disease, as Table 12.1 shows. These include pulmonary fibrosis, pulmonary oedema, pleural effusion, mediastinal widening, pulmonary infiltration and respiratory failure. These drug-induced lung diseases are usually diagnosed only after referral to a chest specialist, after treatments have failed, the symptoms and signs have persisted and the family doctor has become concerned. Unfortunately, in the weeks or months that may have elapsed between presentation and referral, the condition may have worsened, often seriously and sometimes irreversibly – e.g. the truly awful, progressive, avoidable pulmonary fibrosis caused by amiodarone. This is often fatal, after a prolonged terminal phase of extreme dyspnoea. Yet if a knowledgeable family doctor considers this possibility early, in any patient who becomes 'chesty' while taking amiodarone, the fibrosis is often limited and non-progressive.

Please bear this example in mind when studying Table 12.1, and **whenever a patient on regular medication (or a known drug abuser) presents with an unexpected chest problem, consider whether it might be drug induced,** look it up in this book and refer 'on suspicion', without delay.

TABLE 12.1 Drug-induced lung disease. Some of these are uncommon, but if you don't know about them, you may miss important diagnoses

Drug-induced lung disease and the causative drugs	Comments
Asthma	
beta-blockers aspirin Non-steroidal anti-inflammatory drugs Any nebulised medication	Commonly prescribed in family medicine Potentially serious/fatal
Chronic cough	
Angiotensin-converting enzyme inhibitors	Commonly prescribed. Troublesome and may cause non-compliance. Easily recognised
Interstitial pneumonitis/fibrosis	
amiodarone nitrofurantoin	Commonly used in family medicine, fatal if not diagnosed early (*see* Chapter 3 – amiodarone section)
bleomycin busulfan cyclophosphamide	Commonly used in cancer chemotherapy. The family physician is most likely to pick up early pulmonary signs.

(*continued*)

Drug-induced lung disease and the causative drugs	Comments
methysergide (specialist migraine treatment)	A dangerous drug (*see BNF* 4.7–4.2)
phenytoin	Very rare side-effect
Acute hypersensitivity pneumonitis	
infliximab (anti-TNFα) interferon α and β	All increasingly prescribed.
leflunomide	Drug withdrawal recommended
Pulmonary oedema	
Non-cardiogenic	
Aspirin	Commonly prescribed
chlordiazepoxide	Commonly used for alcohol withdrawal
cocaine, especially inhaled 'crack' heroin	Very common drugs of abuse
Cardiogenic beta-blockers	Commonly prescribed negative inotropes
clomiphene	Occurs during ovarian hyperstimulation syndrome
Pleural effusion	
bromocriptine nitrofurantoin	May also cause pulmonary fibrosis
Any drug which induces systemic lupus erythematosus methysergide	May also cause pulmonary fibrosis
Chemotherapeutic agents	May also cause pulmonary fibrosis (see above in table)
Mediastinal widening	
phenytoin	Rare
corticosteroids	Rare
methotrexate	Uncommon
'crack' cocaine	Common in A & E admissions
Pulmonary infiltration	
Without eosinophilia	
amitriptyline azathioprine	Rare – will be diagnosed only with a high 'index of suspicion'
amiodarone	Not uncommon as part of the fatal pulmonary fibrosis caused by amiodarone

(*continued*)

Drug-induced lung disease and the causative drugs	Comments
With eosinophilia	
sulfonamides	Uncommon in family medicine, but not
L-tryptophan	uncommon in chest clinics. Treatment
nitrofurantoin	includes withdrawal of the drug and systemic
penicillins	steroid treatment, often prolonged.
methotrexate	One of many common serious methotrexate ADRs (adverse drug reactions)
'crack' cocaine (inhaled)	Common
paracetamol	Uncommon
ranitidine	
leukotriene antagonists (e.g. montelukast, zafirlukast)	Linked to Churg-Strauss syndrome: unclear if they are an aetiological factor or if they 'unmask' the syndrome
Respiratory failure	
Neuromuscular blockade	May impair neuromuscular transmission
Aminoglycosides (e.g. streptomycin, gentamicin)	(given IM or IV for systemic infections)
Central nervous system depression	
Sedatives	
Hypnotics	
Opioids	Usually occurs in overdosage
Alcohol	
Tricyclic antidepressants	

Acknowledgement: Abridged and annotated from Chesnutt MS and Prendergast TJ. In: Tierney LM, McPhee SJ, Papadakis MA, editors. *Current Medical Diagnosis and Treatment*. 47th ed. New York: Lange/McGraw-Hill; 2008.
With thanks to Dr Cecilia O'Kane, Consultant Respiratory Physician, Belfast City Hospital, for revision of the table.

Every clinician knows that drugs such as amiodarone, methotrexate as a disease-modifying anti-rheumatic drug (DMARD), anti-mitotics or systemic corticosteroids are essential and effective treatments for some disabling or life-threatening conditions, and that it may be difficult to find an adequate alternative. Nevertheless, the potential drug-induced pulmonary harm must be remembered in the presence of chest symptoms, a consultant opinion urgently sought, and the drug withdrawn if necessary.

Finally, apart from drugs causing asthma, pulmonary oedema and respiratory failure, the mechanisms that cause most of these drug-induced pulmonary syndromes are unknown.

13

13

Preventable prescription-related illness caused by patient non-compliance

Twenty years of drug use research across the 'developed' world have shown consistent and worrying evidence of the extent of the non-compliance (or non-adherence) of patients with their prescribed medication – both short-term courses and long-term regimens. In summary, about 20% of patients take their medications (and medicate their children and older dependents) with remarkable precision, gaining maximal benefit as a result. A further 40% take their medicines with varying degrees of imperfection, but well enough to derive therapeutic benefit, although less than if they had self-medicated more precisely. The remaining 40% do not take their prescribed medicines at all, or they take them so badly that they get no benefit what-soever – of these, 15% do not even get their prescriptions dispensed!

The psychological and sociological characteristics of these three groups have been thoroughly studied, and they make interesting background read-ing for the family doctor, aiding a sympathetic understanding of this vagary of human behaviour.[1]

Of more direct relevance to the general practitioner is the realisation that these statistics probably apply to *your* practice, and that 40% of *your* patients gain no benefit from your knowledge, skill, care and effort. The ultimate evidence of the effects of non-compliance is the observation that over 90% of organ transplant rejection (and death) is due to non-compliance with the immunosuppressant regimen. And it has often been reported that up to 70% of asthmatic children admitted to A & E with acute, severe asthma have not been receiving their preventive steroid inhalations regularly. Since the near-abandonment of antipsychotic depot injections, the majority of psychotic patients in the community stop their oral medication, then swing into an acute psychotic episode, with all of its personal and societal sequelae, and then re-start the drug, forgetting that with every relapse the illness deteriorates further and the prognosis worsens.

Non-compliance involves waste. Apart from the waste of the doctors' and pharmacists' time and expertise, and of the NHS budget (on average, about £25 per prescription item), the failure of non-compliant patients to avail themselves of the benefits of modern pharmacology has serious adverse outcomes. Patients with long-term diseases such as diabetes, hypertension, hyperlipidaemia, asthma, rheumatoid arthritis and schizophrenia, who do not take their medicines properly, deteriorate much earlier in life than they need otherwise do, and die earlier – a waste of life itself and of quality of life. Their hospital re-admission rate is much higher than it should be – a vast waste of NHS beds and resources. It is impossible to be precise, but it is estimated that at least £10 billion is wasted each year in the UK, by non-compliance.

It is important for clinicians to know that a subgroup of the 40% of non-compliers are those who take their maintenance regimens intermittently, with gaps of days or weeks, or who 'cherry-pick' their 'favourite' medicines from a regimen of five or more drugs. They do not realise that their prescription was selected to have a balanced, synergistic, long-term effect. This subgroup is at particular risk due to the phenomenon of up-regulation or down-regulation of cell receptors (*see How Drugs Work*, Chapter 6), causing over- or under-physiological compensation when a drug is suddenly stopped. Good examples are anti-hypertensives, SSRI antidepressants and the newer anti-psychotics. The *BNF* clearly advises gradual withdrawal of the latter two drug groups.

For those who wish to know a little more about compliance research findings, there is a short summary at the end of this chapter.

The practical question is 'Can anything be done about non-compliance?' The answer is that much can be done for the majority of the 40% of non-compliers. Many strategies and tactics have been devised, particularly in the USA.[2] Almost all of them have been proved to work for most patients and to improve outcomes, but only for as long as the intervention has continued. When the intervention is stopped, the patients often revert to their previous behaviour.

That being so, here are some of the most effective compliance-enhancing techniques: Many of them involve an extra workload for the prescribing doctor, the nurse, the pharmacist or the carer, or several of them. However, if we are committed to excellence and know that we can substantially improve the care that we give, many of us will be prepared for this extra, paternalistic role of protecting our patients from themselves! If you make that choice, here are some proven and practicable compliance-enhancing methods:

1   *Recognise the problem – diagnose non-compliance.*
    If there is no clinical response, reconsider your diagnosis. If the diagnosis is firm, do not increase the dosage immediately. Ask the patient whether they have any problem in taking the medicines, and to tell you how and how often each drug is to be taken. Then remember that many patients have been shown to lie about their compliance (often to avoid offending you), and check with their pharmacist that their prescriptions have been dispensed and collected. Finally, check whether repeat prescriptions are being requested at approximately the expected intervals.
    When you are reasonably sure that the patient is non-compliant, it is obviously counter-productive to confront them directly.

2   *Ascertain the reason for non-compliance.*
    - Side-effects? Explain that these will often slowly decrease and even disappear.
    - Unsure of the dosage frequency? Explain, write it out and rehearse it at every review.
    - Unable to open the pill bottles? The pharmacist can supply containers with easy-opening caps. But blister packs remain a problem for many.

- Unable to swallow larger tablets or capsules? This is a common problem. Select smaller presentations or prescribe in liquid formulation.
- Unable to remember the regimen? Simplify the regimen as far as possible, and ask the pharmacist to make up a weekly supply in one of the several good dosage aids – this is especially useful for carers.

3 *Educate at every opportunity*, and ask nurses and pharmacists to reinforce the message.

Try to do this in the context of a 'therapeutic contract' between the patient and yourself – a 'concordance.' 'We can do together what neither of us can do alone'. It is a part of the process of teaching and conditioning health behaviour.

4 Try giving the patient a '*drug diary*', to complete daily and bring to you at each review. (This will not suit all patients.)

5 For 'at-risk' patients, *telephonic reminders* have proved very effective, whether by you, the nurse, the pharmacist or the reception staff who deal with repeat prescriptions. Many housebound patients welcome this contact with the outside world.

6 At every opportunity, reassure patients that *they will not become addicted to or dependent on their somatic medications* – this is a major worry for many intelligent lay people, which we doctors are not always aware of.

7 Likewise, reassure patients that *the pure drugs you prescribe are much more effective and usually safer than herbal extracts*, which vary greatly in dosage and may contain dangerous impurities such as the plant's own pesticides, which are potentially toxic.

8 *Nationwide media campaigns*. These have proved very effective in predisposing patients to accept their 'therapeutic contract' with the doctor. However, they need to be repeated fairly frequently, as does all advertising, with new formats for each repetition – cartoons, national celebrities, interviews with 'real people', etc. Unfortunately, the Department of Health has not been particularly consistent about this, and campaigns have been 'few and far between.' However, the doctors, nurses and pharmacists in any region could mount short, frequent campaigns in the local media. These can be very effective – there are always a few good

media communicators in our ranks who would do this well and enjoy it at the same time! Local newspapers, radio and television are glad to get health inputs with a local 'slant', and at no cost!

THE SELF-MEDICATORS: A SPECIAL SUBGROUP OF NON-COMPLIANT PATIENTS

A hundred years ago, the great Canadian physician, Sir William Osler, described humanity as 'the only creature with an intense desire to take medicines!' Humankind has not changed, and the opportunities for self-treating and encouragement to do so are seen in every pharmacy, convenience store and supermarket, not to mention the Internet.

Most people come to no harm in this way, but a small proportion put themselves at serious risk. For example:

1 Patients with any degree of chronic kidney failure may seriously and rapidly worsen their condition by taking aspirin or any NSAID (the author argued at the Committee on Safety of Medicines against a General Sales Licence for NSAIDs, but to no avail. These drugs should not be available in non-pharmacy outlets). Further, NSAIDs interact with numerous commonly prescribed drugs (*see* Chapters 5, 6, 8 and 9 of this book).

2 Patients should be warned not to mix herbal remedies with prescription medicines. The *BNF* (Appendix 1) has 19 entries on drug interactions with St John's wort, and there is a special UK website giving warnings on herbal remedies (www.mhra.gov.uk). Herbals remedies are unstandardised, very impure and not subject to the rigorous safety testing of scientific medicines. It is quite wrong to label them 'complementary and alternative medicines', for they should not be used to complement modern drugs, and they are not a comparable alternative to modern drugs except, perhaps, for the 'worried well' who do not need any medicine, but experience a placebo effect which may be satisfying to them.

All primary care clinicians, doctors, pharmacists and nurses should routinely ask patients who are on maintenance medication whether they are taking any such medicines, or indeed sharing a relative's or neighbour's drugs – all of these things happen!

SUPPLEMENT: SOME TITBITS FROM COMPLIANCE RESEARCH

Non-compliance is of two types – intentional and non-intentional. In the first type, the patient makes a decision not to take the medicines, or to take them as and when they choose, and ignore the directions. In the second type, a variety of factors mitigate against the patient's best intentions.

Intentional non-compliance: the patients' perspectives

1 Some believe that their bodies will self-cure, and do not realise that for most chronic diseases that is not the case.
2 Some doubt the efficacy of modern medicines.
3 Some fear that they will become addicted to their drugs.
4 Some believe that their bodies will develop immunity to long-term treatment.
5 Some dislike 'handing over control' of their bodies and/or minds to medicines (and clinicians) – 'loss of autonomy'.
6 Many imagine that a short course of medicine will cure them of hypertension, diabetes, etc.
7 Many do not comprehend the long-term benefits of maintenance medication, or the risks of having no treatment.
8 Some are worried about side-effects, often with good reason.
9 Some fear 'unnatural, synthetic chemicals', preferring 'natural remedies' without realising the risks that herbals may cause.
10 Some have a completely anti-drug attitude, even to the vaccination of their children.

Apart from the last one, all of these reasons for non-compliance have some underlying rationality, from a lay viewpoint, and all are amenable to repeated, reasoned education in an atmosphere of trust and cooperation. In many cases, the outcome of improved well-being will reinforce compliant behaviour. A significant improvement in self-medication in 50% of non-compliant patients would be a reasonable aspiration.

Unintentional non-compliance

Those whose intended compliance with prescribed medication is seriously hindered include:

1 the confused elderly

2 the forgetful and mentally impaired
3 patients on more than three medicines
4 those with poor eyesight (not helped by the small type on pharmacy bottles) and poor literacy
5 those with arthritis of the hand or wrist and those with inadequate co-ordination, trying to open bottles or express tablets from blister packs
6 those who rely on a carer who doesn't understand or follow the medication schedule.

Great improvements can be achieved in all of these patients with a little effort by the professionals, in contrast to the situation with the intentional non-compliers.

REFERENCES

1 McGavock H, Britten N, Weinman T. *A Review of the Literature on Drug Adherence.* London: Royal Pharmaceutical Society of Great Britain; 1997.
2 Cramer JA, Spilker B. *Patient Compliance in Medical Practice and Therapeutic Trials.* New York: Raven Press; 1991.

14

14

The scientific basis of prescribing for the elderly

Older people account for a growing percentage of the UK population, and for around one-third of primary care workload and prescribing volume. Unfortunately, several studies in European acute geriatric hospital departments have shown that 10–12% of all acute admissions of elderly patients and 18% of elderly deaths are the direct result of prescribed medicines.[1–3] This has been confirmed by a large American study in primary care.[4]

Drug–drug interaction is one of the commonest causes of these admissions, along with patient confusion as to the dosage sequence of several concurrent prescriptions. Such confusion may result in an excessively high dose, particularly of psychotropic drugs.

Hyperkalaemia or hyponatraemia may be caused by chronic diuretic therapy without proper monitoring of blood electrolytes (*see* Chapter 6). Build-up of plasma drug concentrations due to reduced liver and kidney function is common. One or more of the well-known side-effects and interactions of NSAIDs, which were considered in Chapter 5, are common causes of drug-associated illness in the elderly.

Box 14.1 summarises the problem and highlights the fact that 27% of all adverse drug reactions (ADRs) reported to the Committee on Safety of Medicines (CSM) occur in the elderly. It also gives some underlying reasons for this iatrogenic phenomenon.

BOX 14.1 **A large proportion of all adverse drug reactions (ADRs) occur in elderly patients, but these are vastly under-reported**

The problem

Over-65s account for:

- 33% of all prescriptions
- 27% of all reported ADRs; female:male ratio = 2:1
- 15% of the population.

The reasons

Over-65s have:

- decreased salivation and swallowing, protein binding, drug metabolism/ elimination
- altered drug-tissue distribution and drug-tissue responses
- unavoidable polypharmacy (if multiple pathology is present)
- poor medication compliance (often).

THE BIOLOGICAL AGE OF ELDERLY PATIENTS

There is no such thing as a standard prescription for an elderly patient. Therefore it is important to assess the patient's biological age, i.e. are they 'senior athletes' or chronically ill with multiple organ failure and pathology?

Common to all patients over the age of 70 years are the physiological changes of ageing, leading to a gradual reduction in functional reserve in the cardiovascular, respiratory, renal, hepatic, musculoskeletal and central nervous systems, as well as the skin.

Whether a patient's presenting symptoms are due to normal physiological ageing, requiring only reassurance, or to pathology that requires drug treatment, is often a difficult clinical judgement. Good geriatric care is pro-active-preventive.

REDUCED DRUG METABOLISM AND EXCRETION

Tables 14.1 to 14.3 show the essential therapeutic considerations that every prescriber should check-off whenever issuing or repeating a prescription for an older patient. The checklist consists of altered liver and kidney function, nutrition, tissue responses and body composition.

Table 14.1 shows that decreased drug metabolism and excretion are to be expected in older patients, particularly those over the age of 70 years.

TABLE 14.1 The normal ageing process – changes in liver and kidney function

Liver changes	Kidney changes
Decreased blood flow leads to decreased presystemic drug metabolism	The number of nephrons decreases by 6% per decade; although serum creatinine may be normal, older people do have reduced renal function; at 70 years of age, renal function is, at best, 50% of its original maximum. Check the eGFR.
Decreased liver size, microsomal (P450) oxidation and antipyrine clearances lead to decreased hepatic drug metabolism	Decreased glomerular filtration rate and tubular secretion lead to an increased possibility of accumulation of all drugs and metabolites eliminated via the kidneys.
	Note: NSAIDs can accelerate the decline in renal function, particularly in the presence of cardiac failure. Avoid, if possible.

If standard adult doses of many drugs are given to this age group, excessive plasma concentrations will gradually accumulate. The problem is exacerbated by reduced kidney function and a resulting reduction in the ability to excrete drugs and their metabolites. The plasma half-lives of digoxin, lithium and gentamicin are doubled, while that of diazepam may be quadrupled.

The common prescription of NSAIDs for joint pain frequently accelerates this natural decline in renal function by inhibiting renal prostaglandin synthesis, causing tubular ischaemia and retention of sodium and water, which may in turn precipitate or worsen left ventricular failure (*see* Chapter 5).

POOR NUTRITION

It is clearly impossible for nurses, pharmacists and family doctors to be aware of the nutritional status of all their elderly patients, but it is essential to run a mental checklist of nutritional changes whenever prescribing for the elderly (*see* Table 14.2).

TABLE 14.2 The normal ageing process – changes in nutrition and tissue responses

Nutrition changes	Tissue response changes
Vitamins decrease Proteins decrease	Reduction in the number of brain cells increases effects of psychoactive drugs
Nicotine intake unchanged	Reduction in baroreceptor activity increases postural hypotensive effect of drugs
Alcohol intake unchanged	Exaggerated response to anticoagulants; increased risk of gastrointestinal bleeding with NSAIDs

The community dietitian should be asked to survey the nutritional status of less healthy elderly patients on chronic medication, and should be asked about and involved in treatment planning and follow-up.

CHANGES IN TISSUE RESPONSES AND BODY COMPOSITION

The elderly have increased tissue sensitivity to several commonly-needed CNS and cardiovascular drug groups, including the opioid analgesics, the antipsychotics, the antiparkinsonian drugs, the benzodiazepines and digoxin (*see* Table 14.2). The *BNF* clearly indicates which drugs require dosage reduction in the elderly, and some drugs have geriatric formulations – for example, digoxin 62.5 micrograms.

Body composition changes are also important to remember, particularly in patients aged over 75 years, as the reductions in body weight, body water and plasma albumin all conspire to increase the plasma drug concentration and the effect of many medicines (*see* Table 14.3).

SUGGESTIONS FOR RATIONAL GERIATRIC PRESCRIBING

Box 14.2 lists the points to consider when prescribing for elderly patients, particularly if you are considering prescribing a hypnotic, diuretic, NSAID, digoxin, antihypertensive, antiparkinsonian drug, psychotropic drug or warfarin.

BOX 14.2 Points to consider when prescribing for elderly patients

- What is the patient's 'biological age', i.e. is the patient fit for his or her age or should special care be taken with medication, due to overt organ failure?
- Should a low starting dose be used (e.g. calcium–channel blockers, many antidepressants, all benzodiazepines)?
- Does this drug have a small margin of safety (e.g. digoxin, theophylline, lithium, warfarin)?
- What is its route of elimination (e.g. avoid chlorpropamide and glibenclamide in any degree of renal impairment)?
- What interactions may occur with the existing treatment?
- Could the new drug worsen existing pathology (e.g. NSAIDs)?

Box 14.3 lists questions for every medication review, which should be conducted at the time of the patient's annual clinical review and medication review, or more often if indicated.

TABLE 14.3 The normal ageing process – changes in body composition

Changes in body composition	Result
Decreased body weight	Increased effect of standard dose
Decreased body water	Increased plasma concentration of water-soluble drugs
Increased body fat percentage	Decreased plasma concentration of fat-soluble drugs
Decreased plasma albumin	Reduced protein binding

BOX 14.3 Questions to consider when reviewing the current long-term drug treatment of elderly patients

- Is the medication strictly necessary?
- Is it being taken?
- Are there any side-effects?
- Is it having any therapeutic effect?
- Are any of the drugs incompatible?
- Are there signs of drug–drug interaction?

Prescribers should be aware of the common problem of comorbidity in the elderly, leading to unavoidable polypharmacy. This problem is compounded for the prescriber by compelling research-based evidence showing the proven benefits of many drug treatments.

This evidence may indicate that a given patient should be prescribed digoxin, a loop diuretic, an ACE inhibitor, a low-dose cardioselective beta-blocker, warfarin and a statin, for example. The addition of a further drug may incur the risk of a serious ADR, so the decision to prescribe particular treatments and to omit others has to be based on experience and knowledge of the patient, as well as research evidence. Such a decision is perhaps best made in consultation with a geriatrician.

Box 14.4 gives suggested general rules for the prescriber when treating elderly patients. The guidance in Boxes 14.2 to 14.4 could, if followed, improve the health and well-being of your ailing elderly patients, reduce your workload, and greatly reduce the iatrogenic admission rate mentioned at the beginning of this chapter. You may think them worth copying for your practice team.

BOX 14.4 Some rules for prescribers when treating the elderly

- Keep prescribing simple – as few drugs as possible, but polypharmacy may be unavoidable.
- Once- or twice-daily regimens may improve compliance, particularly if associated with mealtimes.
- Encourage a balanced diet – meals on wheels, dietitian, etc.

- Reduce smoking and alcohol intake as much as possible.
- Clear, large labelling is essential.
- Small tablets make swallowing easier as do liquid formulations.
- Avoid modified-release (SR, LA) products unless they are pharmacologi-cally justified. e.g. the short half-lives of nifedipine and diltiazem make them unsuitable for use except in the SR/LA formulation; note that when prescribing maintenance treatment using any SR/LA formula-tion, the same brand name should always be used due to variations in pharmacokinetics between brands.
- Avoid fixed-dose combinations unless they aid compliance.
- Do not use NSAIDs for analgesia only.
- Consider the individual's biological age, not their chronological age.
- Expect adverse drug reactions and interactions in the elderly.
- Cooperate with the patient, the carer, the nurse and the pharmacist, to foster compliance at every opportunity.

CONCLUSION

Prescribing for the elderly is probably the most scientifically demanding area of primary care, but the benefits for the patient and the intellectual satisfaction for the prescriber are well worth the effort.

'At the very least, we should do no harm.'

Hippocrates of Kos

The Royal College of Physicians' report on prescribing for the elderly covers this subject in great detail.[5]

KEY POINTS

- Around 27% of all reported adverse drug events occur in the elderly.
- Around 10–12% of all acute (emergency) hospital admissions in the over-70s are caused by prescribed drugs.
- The anatomical and physiological changes of ageing (listed in this chapter) are partly responsible for these problems.

- The evidence-based co-prescribing of several drugs to treat degenerative disease is another major factor.
- Confusion and poor compliance often contribute.
- The prescriber must select drugs and adjust dosages to take into account reduced liver and kidney function, body composition changes, deficient nutrition and altered tissue responses in the elderly.
- General guidelines are presented in tabular form.

REFERENCES

1 Pirmohamed M, Breckenridge AM, Kitteringham NR *et al*. Adverse drug reactions. *BMJ*. 1998; **316**: 1295–8.
2 Williamson J, Chaplin JM. Adverse drug reactions to prescribed drugs in the elderly: a multicentre investigation. *Age Ageing*. 1980: **9**: 73–80.
3 Ebbeson J, Buajordet I, Erikssen J *et al*. Drug-related deaths in a department of internal medicine. *Arch Intern Med*. 2001; **161**: 2317–23.
4 Huang B, Bachmann KA, Xuming HE *et al*. Inappropriate prescriptions for the aging population of the United States. *Pharmacoepidemiol Drug Safety*. 2002; **11**: 127–34.
5 Royal College of Physicians. *Medication for Older People*. 2nd ed. London: Royal College of Physicians; 1997.

15

15

Clinical quizzes: practical examples from Chapters 1–13

INTRODUCTION

Each quiz relates to one or more chapters from Chapter 1 to 13. The specific chapter, shown in parentheses after the quiz number, contains the full information needed for the solution. All of the quizzes are straightforward, none of them are rare events and if you do not know the solution, as a prescriber you need to study the answer (*see* Chapter 16), and preferably the relevant chapter of the book.

CASE 1 (CHAPTER 1)

A moderately hypertensive 50-year-old man is well controlled at 140/85 on bendroflumethiazide 2.5 mg every morning and 12.5 mg captopril twice daily, both drugs before food. He develops heartburn and buys an antacid from the pharmacist, taking 20 ml four times daily, before meals.

The practice nurse checks his blood pressure a week later and finds it to be 160/92.

Q. What has happened? Specify the mechanism.

CASE 2 (CHAPTER 2)

A 70-year-old, otherwise healthy man developed atrial fibrillation a year ago and is now in sinus rhythm following successful cardioversion, taking warfarin 4 mg daily. His INR is very stable. His only other medication is tadalafil, which he uses once a week, to good effect. His health-conscious wife introduces a glass of grapefruit juice to breakfast every day. A week after starting the grapefruit juice, you receive an emergency house-call and you find the patient:
1 collapsed, with a BP of 90/50
2 with marked subcutaneous bruising.

Q. What has happened? Specify *two* mechanisms.

CASE 3 (CHAPTER 3)

An obese 60-year-old woman with a history of deep venous thrombosis is well stabilised on warfarin, 3 mg daily. She does not require any other medication until she develops knee pain, due to osteoarthritis. She is prescribed naproxen, 250 mg twice daily, which gives her rapid relief. A fortnight later she is admitted to A & E with a gastric bleed which proves difficult to control.

Q. What has happened? Specify *two* mechanisms.

CASE 4 (CHAPTER 4)

A 70-year-old woman has moderate heart failure but is asymptomatic on bendroflumethiazide 2.5 mg, digoxin 62.5 micrograms every morning and ramipril, 1.25 mg twice daily. She develops severe atrial fibrillation, and after failed cardioversion is started on a loading dose of amiodarone, plus the existing medication. Three days later she feels nauseated and weak. On examination, she is found to have a bradycardia of 39/minute, and an ECG shows incomplete heart block. Her BP is 105/25, having been 130/85.

> Q. 1. What has happened (or *not* happened)?
> 2. What should you do in response (that should have been done previously)?

CASE 5 (CHAPTER 4)

The patient in Case 4 settles well, but six months later she attends the practice nurse for an 'elder check-up.' She tells the nurse that she has lost 1½ stone in three months (she had been slightly obese), but feels 'edgy' and snaps at her kindly relatives. The nurse finds her heart rate to be 110 beats/min and regular, and refers her to you.

> Q. 1. What has happened?
> 2. What should you do? Cite the treatment advised in the *BNF* (amiodarone).
> 3. What tests should she have had every six months? (*see BNF*).

CASE 6 (CHAPTERS 4, 9 AND 10)

The patient in Cases 4 and 5 has settled well and continues to take bendroflumethiazide 2.5 mg, digoxin elixir 50 micrograms/ml, 0.5 ml in the morning by dropper, ramipril 1.25 mg twice daily and amiodarone 100 mg twice daily. Six months after the episode in Case 5, she complains of increasing shortness of breath and cough.

> Q. 1. What alarm bells are now ringing?
> 2. What should you do?
> 3. What is the prognosis?

CASE 7 (CHAPTER 5)

A 65-year-old hypertensive man, who survived a myocardial infarction two years ago, is in mild heart failure. He is well controlled on bendroflumethiazide 2.5 mg every morning and lisinopril 20 mg daily, and his BP is 140/90.

He has stopped smoking, and he takes regular exercise. Following some heavy gardening, he develops acute backache and sciatic pain suggestive of an L5-51 disc protrusion. He is prescribed rest and diclofenac 25 mg three times daily. Within a week his lumbago and sciatica have settled, but he attends you complaining of ankle swelling. On examination you find that he has indeed developed ankle oedema and his blood pressure has risen to 165/100.

Q. 1. What has happened? Specify *two* mechanisms.
   2. What action should you take, in terms of prescribing?

CASE 8 (CHAPTER 6)

A retired labourer in moderate heart failure has been taking furosemide, an ACEI and spironolactone daily for the past nine months. He misses three review appointments. One evening he collapses at home and the paramedics find a low blood pressure and a very abnormal ECG trace, but no ECG evidence of infarction.

Q. What may be the cause of his collapse?
   Sequel: In A & E, his electrolytes show profound hyponatraemia and moderate hypokalaemia – a life-threatening metabolic emergency.

Q. What combined renal effects of his medication have caused this?
   Suggestion: Ask your local A & E consultant how often they encounter this problem.

CASE 9 (CHAPTER 8)

A 55-year-old man, who was asthmatic as a teenager, is in severe heart failure as a result of untreated hypertension (he had refused both specialist referral and medication). In hospital, he was prescribed a low-dose selective β_1 beta-blocker in an attempt to control his refractory CHF. Within hours, he developed acute severe asthma, due to the effect of the selective beta-blocker on his bronchiolar β_2-receptors (selectivity is only relative). During emergency treatment, he does not respond adequately to nebulised salbutamol.

Q. What is the reason for his non-response? Specify the mechanism.

CASE 10 (CHAPTER 9)

A patient with bipolar illness is well stabilised on lithium, and attends the local lithium clinic monthly. He develops a dental root abscess and is prescribed metronidazole 400 mg, 8-hourly, for seven days. On the fifth day, he develops tremor, unsteadiness and slurring of his speech.

Q. 1. What has happened? Specify the mechanism.
2. How might it have been avoided?

CASE 11 (CHAPTER 9)

A 50-year-old woman with type 2 diabetes is well controlled on diet, exercise and gliclazide 160 mg daily. She develops severe oral thrush and is prescribed miconazole gel, retained in the mouth four times daily after meals, then swallowed. On the fifth day she develops her first 'hypo' (hypoglycaemic reaction) in several years. She swallows several glucose tablets and telephones the diabetic nurse specialist.

Q. 1. What caused the hypoglycaemia? State the mechanism.
2. What advice should she be given (a) now and (b) 48 hours after her oral thrush has cleared?

CASE 12 (CHAPTER 10)

A young man is a 'heavy social drinker' but has no other health problems. He is prescribed griseofulvin tablets, 500 mg daily, for acute tinea capitis. After 24 hours' treatment he goes out for an evening 'with the lads.' By the third drink, he feels nauseated, vomits, feels his face flushing and has a severe headache. His friends take him to A & E – quite rightly.

Q. 1. What has caused this attack?
2. What is its 'generic' name?
3. What other commonly used drugs may cause it?

CASE 13 (CHAPTERS 9 AND 13)

A 33-year-old woman, a teacher, who is married and has 'completed her family', is on a low-dose oral contraceptive. Feeling tired and depressed at the end of a difficult term, she takes a friend's advice and begins a course of St John's wort. With a combination of the school holiday, the placebo effect and the mild antidepressant effect of the hypericin and hyperforin in the St John's wort, she feels much better. A month later, she discovers to her horror that she is pregnant.

Q. Why has her oral contraceptive failed? Specify the mechanism.

16

16

Answers to clinical quizzes

INTRODUCTION

The following answers are brief summaries. For more detail, see the relevant chapter(s).

CASE 1 (CHAPTER 1)

A chemical reaction has occurred in the patient's stomach, between aluminium, magnesium or calcium ions and the captopril molecules. This has de-activated the captopril or rendered it incapable of absorption from the small intestine, resulting in inadequate plasma concentrations of the antihypertensive drug.

A similar reaction occurs with several common antibiotics and antifungals, some anti-epileptics, some anti-malarials, an antiviral, the bisphosphonates, digoxin, oral iron and lansoprazole, leading to the relevant therapeutic failure.

Note: If the drugs are taken before food and the antacid after food, this effect should not occur. It is dependent on the presence of antacid in the stomach at the same time as the drug.

CASE 2 (CHAPTER 2)

A 250-ml glass of grapefruit juice or half a grapefruit increases the absorption from the jejunum of many drugs, including warfarin and the erection enhancers. For the mechanism (which is interesting), *see* Chapter 2.

Other drugs whose plasma concentrations are increased by grapefruit juice include the calcium-channel blockers, several immunosuppressants, several antivirals, atorvastatin, amiodarone, sertraline and buspirone.

Note: The glass of grapefruit juice has an effect which lasts 24 hours – any susceptible medicine taken during that time will have increased intestinal absorption.

CASE 3 (CHAPTER 3)

This is a 'double whammy.' The NSAID has caused gastric erosion and bleeding, while the warfarin has reduced the body's clotting response, resulting in profuse haemorrhage.

If any NSAID, including COX-2 inhibitors, must be given to an anticoagulated patient, it may be wise to add a proton pump inhibitor.

Macrolides (erythromycin, etc.), quinolones (ciprofloxacin, etc.) antifungals, sulphonylureas, SSRIs, amiodarone and phenytoin all potentiate warfarin and increase the risk of bleeding.

CASE 4 (CHAPTER 4)

This patient has developed digoxin toxicity. Plasma digoxin levels increased because the amiodarone substantially reduced the metabolism of digoxin in the liver and its renal clearance. The dose of digoxin should usually be halved if amiodarone is to be added (*BNF*).

Response: In consultation with a cardiologist, withdraw the digoxin and reduce the dose of amiodarone.

CASE 5 (CHAPTER 4)

1 Of the many adverse side-effects of amiodarone, one of the best known is the development of thyrotoxicosis.
2 The amiodarone should be withdrawn (at least temporarily) and treatment with carbinazole may be necessary. Hypothyroidism may also occur – treat by replacement therapy.
3 Thyroid function, liver function and serum electrolytes should be checked before treatment with amiodarone and six-monthly thereafter.

CASE 6 (CHAPTERS 4 AND 12)

1 One of the most devastating adverse effects of amiodarone is pulmonary fibrosis. If this is not detected early and the drug stopped, it is irreversible and often fatal.
2 Immediate referral to a specialist respiratory unit is required.
3 If the family doctor detects the problem early (from systematic questioning about dyspnoea and cough at each review) and stops the amiodarone, the fibrosis may be limited.

CASE 7 (CHAPTER 5)

Two of the ten adverse side-effects of all NSAIDs are:
1 They reduce the effectiveness of all antihypertensives.
2 They worsen congestive heart failure both by increasing plasma fluid volume and by a direct negative inotropic effect on the myocardium.

Hence this patient's higher blood pressure and loss of control of his heart failure.

The NSAID should be withdrawn.

Comment: NSAIDs are such useful anti-rheumatic drugs when inflammation is present (as in an acute disc lesion), or in rheumatoid arthritis, that it may be difficult to avoid their use. So long as the prescriber is fully aware of the NSAID side-effects specified in Chapter 5, it may often be possible to achieve a therapeutic compromise.

CASE 8 (CHAPTER 6)

Rationale: Furosemide causes overall loss of K+, Mg^{2+} and Ca^{2+}. ACEIs cause Na+ loss and some K+ retention. Spironolactone causes Na+ loss and some K+ retention.

Overall result in this patient: Profound hyponatraemia and moderate hypokalaemia – a life-threatening metabolic emergency.

See Chapter 6 for a fuller explanation.

CASE 9 (CHAPTER 8)

Most clinicians know that even a small dose of any beta-blocker may precipitate acute severe asthma in a patient with a past history. What is not always remembered is that even selective β_1-blockers have some blocking action on β_2-receptors in the bronchial tree. As well as precipitating asthma, this beta-blockade prevents access of the bronchodilators salbutamol or terbutaline to the β_2-receptors – a double jeopardy for the patient.

CASE 10 (CHAPTER 9)

1 The patient is lithium toxic and at serious risk. The metronidazole has inhibited the metabolism of the lithium, leading to toxic concentration of lithium. Admit him to A & E immediately, with your presumptive diagnosis.
2 He should have been prescribed high-dose amoxicillin, or erythromycin, if penicillin allergic.

CASE 11 (CHAPTER 9)

1 Significant amounts of miconazole are absorbed systemically from the oral gel. Several of the 'azole' antifungals increase the plasma concentration of sulphonylureas, causing a moderate hypoglycaemia.
2 Reduce the dose of gliclazide for 24 hours, and then resume at the previous dose. Stop the miconazole and prescribe an antiseptic mouthwash. Check for the source of the candidal infection.

CASE 12 (CHAPTER 10)

1 The griseofulvin has caused an 'antabuse' reaction with the alcohol (*see* Chapter 10).
2 The 'antabuse' reaction.
3 The cephalosporins, the sulphonamides, nitrofurantoin, metronidazole, isoniazid, the nitrates and sulphonylureas can also precipitate the same reaction, which increases in severity as the intake of alcohol increases.

CASE 13 (CHAPTERS 9 AND 13)

St John's wort causes increased activity (induction) of the liver enzymes which metabolise many other drugs. It therefore reduces the contraceptive effect of oestrogens by accelerating their metabolism. The *BNF* warns: 'avoid concomitant use.'

Index